MW00973666

Disclaimer:

The information in this book is not meant as a substitute for the medical advice of physicians and/or mental health professionals. The reader should consult with a licensed medical practitioner and never use the information in this book to diagnose or treat any disease or disorder. Medications should always and only be taken under a doctor's advice and supervision. Information in this publication is not meant as advice but only as recommendations to be utilized at your own risk. The author or publisher does not assume any liability for the use, inability to use, or misuse of information contained in this publication.

Reading and implementing ANY of the ideas and recommendations in this book does not guarantee that expected results will be manifested.

The author or publisher will not be held responsible for any errors or omissions that may be found.

Note: Some of the names in this book have been changed to protect the privacy of individuals.

Dedication

This book is dedicated to my loving husband Scott and my two amazing and beautiful daughters, all of whom patiently supported me, gave valuable input, and stood by me throughout this exciting endeavor. I also want to dedicate this book to my mom for her help and support in the writing of this book, and for her wonderful example of how to parent with infinite love, patience, and wisdom.

Table of Contents

Intro Letter

Dear Parent(s),

Welcome to the "The Complete and Practical Guide to Raising Your ADD Child to Success." I am grateful you are here, and I believe you have made one of the best decisions of your life for ensuring the success of your child.

Before we dig in, let me just explain briefly how I will refer to certain things throughout this book, for the sake of simplicity. I will refer to your child with ADHD as "your child" and as "he" and "him."

I will also use the pronoun "I" when referring to me, but often this includes my husband, who so faithfully and determinedly walked alongside me in our journey with our own child and in the writing of this book.

When speaking of your child's teacher, I will use the pronouns "she" and "her."

Also, I will use the term ADD interchangeably with ADHD. I am confident that this book will be useful for those with children who have ADHD of the hyperactive, inattentive or combination type.

I do not specifically address severe symptoms that sometimes accompany ADD, such as social anxiety disorder, ODD, etc., although many of these ideas and strategies will undoubtedly be useful for those children as well.

Now with that out of the way (thank you for hanging in there with me), let's turn the page and get started!

Sincerely,

Karen Murphy

INTRODUCTION

Hello again...

My name is Karen Murphy. Thank you for the opportunity to help you with what I believe to be one of the MOST important things you will ever do ... help your child succeed!

Before we dive in, please allow me to give you some background on myself that many of you will find important and relatable.

I am the very proud parent of a child with ADD. Our daughter, Tena (pronounced Tina), was diagnosed at age 8 with ADHD inattentive (basically ADHD without the H as I like to call it). Tena had some of the classic symptoms:

- Trouble staying on task

- Unable to remember more than 2 things at a time

- Very easily distracted

- Difficulty reading and testing

- Weak working memory.

- Didn't catch the meaning of jokes and sarcasm

She hated to read. She hated it so much she would say to me that she could not go into the library with me because the library gives her a headache. She didn't even want to be around books!

I tried numerous things to help her:

- Natural Supplements

- Pharmaceutical medication

- Changes in her diet

- Biofeedback

- Several different schools

- Private tutoring

- Learning centers

- Brain training

- A bunch of other stuff!

With a few, there was some success, but with others – none.

And so it was with many of these "experiments." I fondly call Tena my "guinea pig" because I tried so many different ways to help her.

So here we are, at the writing of this book, 11 years after Tena's initial diagnosis.

Where is she now?

- A freshman in college

- Great friends in her life

- Working two part time jobs

- Volunteering once a week in the church nursery

- The favorite of many of her teachers and friends' parents

- Great work ethic

- A joy to be around

This is the result of a lot of hard work on the part of Tena, myself and her dad. But we can't take ALL the credit. We did get some outside help, some of which actually worked. I'll get into that in chapter 10. But I guarantee you that the changes we made at home and at school definitely played a large part in her success.

And to be sure, Tena is not cured. She's not perfect. There are still struggles and obstacles that she faces every day.

If you ask her too many things at once, she gets overwhelmed. She will ask me to stop and ask one thing at a time.

She gets confused trying to keep up with her bank account or making change. Small detail oriented tasks are difficult.

Words that are too close together on a page are difficult for her to read and interfere with her comprehension.

Trying to write inside narrow lines is hard. To this day she will not use college ruled notebook paper. She will only use wide ruled.

But she is doing so much better than she was. She has learned adaptive measures to help herself, like the wide ruled paper, for example. She makes lists, she keeps an agenda. She recognizes her weaknesses and has learned how to work with these challenges.

She's self-confident and self-assured. She's determined to do her best in college, in her job, in her LIFE, no matter what it takes.

I believe I have succeeded in helping Tena, despite her ADD and learning disabilities, to have:

Stellar Success in school, at home, in life

And that is exactly what this book will help you to achieve with your child as well.

Your child is special in so many ways. Not "special" in the sense that he is less than "normal" or deficient in some way, but special because he is an amazing person, with incredible capabilities and talents. You will discover how many of these "disabilities" he has are actually strengths and gifts and you'll learn how to foster and nurture these gifts to help your child succeed.

I realize that your child may have ADD symptoms that are more severe or less severe than Tena's. Your child may have serious behavior problems, severe learning disabilities or even other "disorders" such as ODD (Oppositional Defiant Disorder), all of which can accompany ADD.

I don't claim that this book will cure or fix these "disorders", but I am confident that no matter what the challenges or diagnosis, no matter how old or young your child is, there are elements in this book that WILL help.

As you may have already discovered, information out there on raising a child with ADD is enormous, and you can literally spend hours, days, years, reading and learning excellent strategies and techniques on helping your child succeed.

But as I quickly learned, after spending hours, days and months reading this stuff, the end result was not that I learned how to help my daughter, but that I got overwhelmed to the point where I wasn't much use to her at all.

The problem for me was TOO MUCH INFORMATION! I was overwhelmed. Where do I start? What will work, what won't? How do I do ALL OF THIS STUFF?

Thus, "The Complete Practical Guide..." was born! I realized that what I needed was a short compilation of the best and most practical information out there. I did not need an anatomy lesson on the brain or details about every medication. Later maybe, but at that time I just needed help with what I could do and do NOW!

And that's exactly what this book does. It combines the best of the best, including what I've gathered from books and articles, my personal experience and the experiences of friends and family. I've also included advice and insight I've been privileged to receive directly from experts who work one on one with these special children.

Now don't get me wrong. You can never really have too much information. However, when you are trying to implement what you learn while you're learning it, and you're learning 5 million things at once, and some of it is so technical it takes a rocket scientist to understand...

Paralysis sets in!

You do nothing. You can't think.

At least that's what happened to me.

Try this: Read this book and start implementing the ideas and strategies. You'll be encouraged by the results that you see. But also, now or later, whatever works for you, read other books. Read everything you can get your hands on! Talk to other parents, talk to experts in the field. At the end of this book, where I list my sources, I will also have some additional resources for you such as websites for schools specializing in learning differences, yahoo groups, therapies, and organizations all centered on ADHD. Check them all out. You will find valuable information and valuable support.

CHAPTER 1

What is ADD and how will it Affect My Child's Life?

First let me say that I'm not going to venture very deeply into all the technical and medical information on brain function and what causes ADD. Most of what we need to know as parents is that our child is struggling and how to bring him to a place of success in life.

There are conflicting answers to the question of what causes ADD.

Some studies have shown one thing, while similar studies do not collaborate the findings. But there are a number of studies that have been done with similar findings across the board that conclude that ADD can be due to:

- Genetics

- Deficiency in the neurotransmitter serotonin

- Reduced blood flow to the frontal part of the brain

- Lower level of brain's electrical activity seen on EEG than on children without ADD.

- Trauma to the frontal part of the brain

- Thinner, less developed tissue in the brain area (2007 research from the National Institute of Mental Health) This can cause delayed brain development resulting in development being approximately 2-3 years behind average)

Boys are more likely to be diagnosed with the hyperactive form of ADHD while girls are typically diagnosed ADHD inattentive.

What are some of the symptoms of a person with ADD?

- Has difficulty paying attention and staying on task

- Makes careless mistakes

- Does not seem to listen when spoken to

- Has trouble changing tasks or handling changes in routine

- Disorganized

- Forgetful, loses things

- Distracted easily

- Blurts things out without thinking

- Habit of touching things and people

- Impulsive behavior and fidgety

- Over sensitive and easily frustrated

- Highly energetic (hyperactive)

Wow, this sounds like most kids! You're right. Let me ask you a question: How many kids do you know that:

- Can't sit quietly and listen to a 30 min. lecture?

- Try to leave the dinner table to go finish his video game or go outside to play?

- Loses things

- Forgets half of what his mom just told him to do?

- Has a lot of energy?

My guess is that you'll answer something like, "All the kids I know are like that!"

Probably pretty close to the truth.

The ADD child is a regular kid with many "typical" childhood behaviors and traits magnified 2, 3 or 10 times.

Ok, great. So how do I know then if my child is ADD or if he is just being a regular kid or going through some sort of phase?

Great question! You may or may not know for sure that your child has ADD but since you are reading this book I'm going to assume that you strongly suspect it.

When a child exhibits several of these traits (many of them stronger in intensity than in the average child), causing him to be strongly impaired in his work, activities and/or social interactions, he goes from "typical kid" to a kid with ADD. It is typical child traits gone haywire or "typical on steroids" you might say.

Many children with ADD have at least one type of learning disability in math, reading or science. Many have problems w/working memory, auditory processing or listening comprehension. Some ADD children may also have ODD (oppositional defiant disorder), anxiety, Tourette's syndrome or some other accompanying disorder.

A lot of children with ADD struggle in academics. They may have trouble getting work done in a timely manner, or understanding what they read or figuring out math problems. You (and he) may think that he just isn't very smart or that maybe his IQ is a little on the lower end.

But it really has nothing to do with IQ. In fact, a 2009 Yale University study showed that 75% of kids with ADHD had a high IQ (scores of 120 and higher.) However, due to the symptoms caused by their ADD, they had significant impairment in their cognitive abilities.

The good news is, your kid is likely much smarter than you or he may think! He just needs some extra help. Using the strategies and ideas in this book will help him to reach his true potential.

Behavior

Negative behavior can be very prevalent in a child with ADD. Some of it is just the ADD. He is disrupting the class because of his hyperactivity; he is not doing his homework because he forgets.

Negative behavior is sometimes a "side effect" of ADD. These children often have a low self-concept due to the failures and negative experiences they have because of their ADD (such as poor grades or teasing by classmates). It can be difficult for them to articulate these feelings so, they instead, act them out.

Bad behavior is often the result of bad feelings. It is so important to talk with your child and try to find the reason behind his behavior. If you help him sort through his feelings and try to get to the bottom of it, you have a head start in working on a solution.

It is so painful for a parent to witness their child struggling. You want the best for him. You want him to have a "normal" childhood but he just isn't. He's not being invited to sleepovers, not talking on the phone with friends, and not making decent grades in school. He may be friendless, failing, bored, lonely. His self-esteem and self-confidence is suffering. He feels out of control, inferior. Your home life may be very chaotic. He's not getting along with you or with his siblings.

No matter how hard you try, nothing seems to help. You feel, well,

helpless.

You are not helpless however, and this is not hopeless. There are literally hundreds of options out there to help you and your child.

This diagnosis is not a death sentence. It is not the end of the world. On the contrary!

This is the beginning of a new lease on life for you and your child; a time to start fresh and do things differently. There is a light at the end of the tunnel. These seemingly never-ending problems may actually have a solution!

You now know that your child's behavior is not due to bad parenting. It is not your fault!

Try to relax in the fact that if you know he has ADD, you can now do something about it.

Key #1: ADD is for real

Unfortunately, there are those skeptics out there who think ADD is some kind of fabricated disorder or an excuse for less than attractive behavior or abilities.

You may even be one of those skeptics.

Truly, ADD is for real. Don't let anyone tell you otherwise - that it is over diagnosed, or your kid just needs more structure.

ADHD is recognized by The American Psychiatric Society as a medical diagnosis. It is listed in the DSM (Diagnostic and Statistical Manual of Mental Disorders.) It is definitely a real disorder and your child may have it.

When Tena was diagnosed, in some ways it was a relief. I finally realized it wasn't my fault. I wasn't some lousy, dufus mom who didn't know what I was doing. There were reasons for Tena's struggles and ways to help her.

If you suspect your child has ADD and want to know for sure, please get him tested. Find a reputable doctor, psychologist, psychiatrist or counselor that can do these tests for you. Remember, some specialists can be quick to diagnosis ADHD. Please do your research and ask other people's advice on whom to see. Your specialist should be very thorough, first acquiring all the information and history on your child regarding what you have seen that makes you suspect ADHD. When they test, they should do one test at a time to see if there are any red flags warranting more tests. Your specialist may discover ADHD and also other disorders that sometimes accompany ADHD, such as learning disabilities, auditory processing issues, and problems with working memory.

We didn't get Tena tested until she was 9 years old and in the 4th grade. I started to notice some signs of it a couple of years before that, but I just attributed it to her being a kid.

When Tena was in the second grade, the signs became more apparent.

At this time Tena went to a private school. I volunteered in her classroom once a week reading with a group of kids. The kids would take turns reading from the book, and then I would ask questions at the end. Tena could read very well. She knew how to sound out the words and she was pretty fluent.

When the questions came at the end of the story, most kids would be fairly accurate in their answers, but not Tena. I would ask her a question relating to what we just read and she would come up with something that had almost nothing to do with the question. It was so perplexing. For example, the story might have said something like this:

"Mrs. Ray raised puppies in her home but she didn't like to sell them because she loved them too much.

Question: Why did Mrs. Ray not like to sell her puppies?

Tena: She liked to cook in her new kitchen.

Total disconnect. Maybe the lady did like to cook, maybe she had a new kitchen, but that had nothing to do with her selling puppies. The reason behind this disconnect, I later found out, was ADD combined with other learning disabilities - in her case, working memory problems, slower auditory processing and listening comprehension issues.

When that school year ended, I took Tena out of school and homeschooled her, thinking she just needed some one on one attention and this reading problem would be solved.

Not exactly.

The problems extended far beyond just reading. Tena didn't understand directions well, wasn't learning her math facts and was having trouble doing any math that required more than one step (such as carrying over in subtraction). She made careless mistakes like putting an answer in the wrong place or adding instead of subtracting. These were all due to her ADD with a helping of learning disabilities on the side.

Other things I noticed: forgetfulness and disorganization. I remember a time when Tena's teacher, Ms. Ragen, told me that Tena had not been turning in her homework assignments. I knew she did them, because I always made sure her homework was done, whether she needed my help or not. Even to this day I do tend to be a bit of a micromanager!

I then asked Tena about her homework.

She told me she always brought her homework in to school and turned it in. Well, Ms. Ragen and I could not figure out what could have happened to her homework until one day Ms. Ragen looked in Tena's cubby!

Her cubby, the little box where she kept all her stuff she did each day and kept her pencils, papers, artwork, etc., was full of papers crumpled up inside.

When Ms. Ragen went through these papers, lo and behold, she found the assignments from the past few weeks. Tena knew she brought them, which she did, but they never made it to the teacher's desk.

You may be wondering if this type of thing will last forever. Can a person outgrow ADD?

Symptoms can fade significantly but research does not support that it goes away entirely. A child can "outgrow" ADD to a point where it doesn't impair him nearly as much as it impaired him as a child. Studies show that there is often a 3-year delay in the brain development of a person with ADD. Therefore, over time there could be significant lessening of symptoms, even to the point where they are virtually gone, but not necessarily non-existent.

Studies do show that about 60% of children with ADD retain some symptoms through adulthood.

This is not good news. Adult ADD can be very damaging to a person's well being if they haven't learned coping and adaptation skills to deal with it early in life.

Make sure your child learns methods and strategies so he can use them on his own as an adult.

We once had a neighbor who was about 40 years old and had ADD.

What did the life of Jason look like?

- He did not keep up with the bills, and they lost power and gas service at least twice in the two years they lived next door.

- He had traffic tickets he forgot to pay. One day he got pulled over for something unrelated and ended up going to jail.

- He could not hold down a job and his wife supported him, resulting in a turbulent 14 year marriage that ended in divorce.

- When his wife lost her job they were evicted from their house. He neglected to address the non-payment notices that were on his door every week for three weeks.

I'm not trying to scare you, but ADD can be detrimental to your child's future.

You cannot wait until if and when your child outgrows his ADD symptoms!

He needs help NOW. If you work with your child throughout his young life, you will be able to teach him the adaptive behaviors that will help him through the challenges that ADD poses for him. If he does not learn these and he still retains the symptoms as an adult, it will interfere with his adult life. Adults with ADD often suffer from depression, anxiety and substance abuse, and they struggle with success in relationships and career.

It may seem like its light years away but one day, before you know it, he will be an adult. Give him that gift and teach him how to overcome the challenges on his own. Help him on his way to a successful adult life!

CHAPTER 2

MINDSET MATTERS

So, what is that phrase in the title of this book - "Stellar Success in school, at home, in life?"

Is this a joke? "My kid? I don't think so!" Well, I'm here to tell you, YES, your kid! Successful - in all areas of life.

Please know that this is absolutely possible. You may have had so many bad experiences, so much trial and error, so much frustration, so many tears, that you think this just cannot be. But I'm here to tell you it can be done. It has been done. And not only by me, but by hundreds if not thousands of parents who have implemented many of these methods you're about to learn.

Discovering these methods has been life changing for my family, and it will be for you as well. It's time to believe for the best.

Before I go on, let me say that I personally do not like the term "disorder" when it comes to describing ADD. Your child has some brain differences (and I am not trying to be politically correct here) and yes, they can cause impairment in learning and behavior.

Understand that the way your child thinks about his diagnosis is ultra-important. When all the problems with Tena peaked to where we took her for testing, it was a relief to all of us that there was a name and a reason for it.

Make sure your child does not look at it as some kind of disease and that he is doomed to failure. The danger of labeling something as a disorder or disability is that it gives the impression that change and improvement are not possible.

As parents it is our job to help them have the right perception of their "differences."

Did you know that some of the most accomplished people in the world have ADD or were thought to have had it?

To name a few:

- Albert Einstein

- Vincent Van Gogh

- Wolfgang Mozart

- Henry Ford

- Christopher Columbus

- Jim Carrey

- John F. Kennedy

- Justin Timberlake

- Whoopie Goldberg

- Agatha Christie

- Michael Phelps

It's time to stop worrying that your child will amount to nothing or that he'll spend most of his life behind bars. His potential is limitless and you need to believe it.

Belief, Positivity, Praise...These are not just some New Age cliché's or some hokey feel-good answer to life's problems. The mind is a powerful thing. We'll look at each of these as we go through this chapter.

First, let's talk about belief:

Countless studies have shown that people generally perform the way they are expected to perform. If a person thinks or believes a certain way, then eventually that belief will manifest itself.

When I was a kid, I tended to be a little uncoordinated. My best friend, with whom I spent almost every day from the time I was 11 until I was 18, would repeatedly say to me, "you're such a klutz!" I can tell you, every time I was with her I became more of a klutz than the last time, and even when not with her I seemed to become klutzier by the day.

To give you a visual, I tripped a lot, stubbed my toe, got my fingers caught in doors. Even weird things would happen to me like while sitting outside I would suddenly feel a warm moist plop on my head and discover that the bird above me just relieved himself!

I believed that I was a klutz, and so I became one.

When you believe something, you will behave in a way that reflects that belief. If you don't believe, you will behave in a way that reflects that unbelief.

Let's say you don't think your child will ever get a particular math problem. You will probably do one of three things:

- Gloss over the problem and not even let him try it.

- Tell him this one is especially hard and you'll skip it or go back to it later.

- Try it for 5 seconds and see that he doesn't get it, and then give up.

You might not even realize you did it. Even though it may be subconscious on your part, your child can tell that you don't think he can do this problem. These ways of "handling" a difficult math problem can and do kill a kid's confidence. When you do this, he will know you don't have faith in him; therefore, he won't have faith in himself.

Too often, we parents see the limitations of our children and not the potential.

One of the most incredible stories I've heard about belief taking over and trumping weakness or disability, was a story I read in the book "Think and Grow Rich" by Napoleon Hill. The book was written in 1939 but is still relevant today and is still a top seller in the realm of the wealth-building industry.

Mr. Hill's son was born without the natural apparatuses needed for hearing. All his doctors said he would likely be a deaf-mute for life. He did indeed show the symptoms of a severely hearing impaired child, but he could hear slightly. He did not attempt to speak at the age when children normally begin that process.

Mr. Hill made a decision that his son would not remain a deaf-mute but that he would hear and lead a "normal" life. He made sure he transferred that desire and belief to his son. To make a long story short, this belief and desire turned into persistence on his and his son's part to do what it took, and eventually that deaf-mute child attended college and later became a spokesperson for an innovative hearing device. He sold thousands of these devices and became a very successful businessman.

Ok, so do you now know your child can be successful? Great...

Make sure HE knows it too.

Next:

Don't belittle your child!

Really Karen? You think you need to tell me that? Who would ever belittle their kid?

You.

Most likely, in some way, shape or form, either out right or subtly, you do it.

I did it.

As you may have noticed, kids with ADD are very good at belittling themselves. "I'm stupid" or "no one likes me" are common phrases of the ADD child. Don't add your own negativity to the mix.

Instead, take advantage of these negative statements he makes about himself. Turn them around. Help him see that what he said is ABSOLUTELY NOT TRUE!!

For example, the "I'm stupid" remark. Think of some accomplishment, excellent grade he made on an assignment or difficult book he read.

"Someone who is stupid could never have gotten a B on that homework assignment. That math was really difficult."

"I know you think no one likes you, but you and Kyle are good buddies. He likes you. You are a very likable person."

ALWAYS, ALWAYS remind him of the positives in his life. Do your best to constantly show him positives about himself. He is an awesome, valuable and precious human being. Help him see that!

Regular positive input is crucial. I implore you, be CAREFUL with what you input into your child. Those negative comments you make are going to stick like krazy glue in your kid's brain for a long time to come.

And know this:

It's not just your words.

It's the way you subtly shake your head or roll your eyes, the long sighs you let out or the slumping of your shoulders. Your kid sees it; he feels it. Never show frustration as long as you can help it (I know it's hard. As the saying goes, "Never let them see you sweat."

Your child is already frustrated enough with himself. Seeing you get frustrated or losing confidence will cause your child to feel even more frustrated and hopeless.

"Too late Karen," you say. "I've already done that" or "I do that all the time."

It's ok...start NOW. Don't beat yourself up. We've all done it, and it's not too late.

I not so fondly remember reading with Tena when she was young, being worse than negative. I would ask her questions about a passage, and she could not see the answers even though they were right there word for word.

Me: Do I have to read it AGAIN!?? Listen this time! Are you paying attention? The answer is RIGHT HERE!!

Heavy sighs, angry voice.

I would literally feel sick to my stomach after one of these episodes, and Tena would be in tears, but I couldn't seem to control myself. I made her feel stupid, and at time I was so frustrated, I frankly don't think I cared. Sad but true.

I crushed Tena's spirit. We parents are experts at that. Some of our child's teachers are experts at that. You never want to crush their spirit. You want to lift them up.

After several of these episodes, I finally took myself and Tena to counseling. It was then that it was suggested she be tested. Our counselor assured me that Tena would not purposely do this, and I knew he was right.

Watch out for that negative energy, subtle or not so subtle. Know that patience, confidence, and faith in him will pay off in the end.

Remember I said that the ADD kid is just a regular kid? It's true and chances are whether or not you have ADD yourself, you may have had behaviors, problems and weaknesses similar to your child's.

Share these with him!

I always had a lot of trouble with math - not my forte - and had to get tutoring, even in basic high school math classes. Homework was frustrating and usually brought me to tears.

Just sharing this with Tena helped her to feel that she wasn't alone and that she wasn't so different. Other people struggle with these things too. And there's obviously hope. My math isn't great, but I overcame the worst of it, and she can too.

Alright. I think you get the positive-negative input stuff.

So let's go on to praise.

Sometimes it's hard to find things you can praise your child about. Things can be going so badly ... behavior is poor, grades are poor, temper flares, inappropriate behavior abounds.

But your child has praiseworthy traits! Find them and focus on them. If you can only think of one right now, capitalize on it!

I currently mentor a child in a nearby public school. We'll call him Steven. He is in first grade and has ADHD, WITH the "H." He is a very sweet child, but he has trouble sitting still. When he gets up to do something, for example, he leaves the table to throw something away and he's gone for 5 minutes because he gets distracted and starts doing other things. I have to repeatedly tell him to return to the table. If I keep him busy enough, he does better, but the minute he's "free" for even a second, he's off! He has some anger issues and gets in trouble at school and sometimes gets in fights. Once he was suspended for a day, because he told a classmate he was going to cut him with a knife, tie him up and throw him in the dumpster.

Steven is very smart though. And he loves his mom and talks about her and misses her while he's at school. He loves his siblings.

For a while, these were the only truly positive things I could see in him.

Therefore, I praised him for those things. I told him how impressed I was with a math problem he did or how I loved the picture he drew I told him how lucky his mom is to have a son that loves her and how proud she must be of him.

Praise your child for things he can control. Don't just say, "you're so smart," but instead, be specific. For example, tell him how he read something well and with such enthusiasm. If he does small, kind deeds or openly shows affection, tell him how it makes your day when he gives you those hugs or how he makes people happy by doing special little things for them.

Is he good at a sport, an instrument, building Legos?

Remember to affirm that to him, praise him for that great hit in baseball or the way he is persistent in practicing the piano. Some more practical examples:

- He hasn't touched his brother or fiddled with an object for a full 10 minutes one morning. Tell him how proud you are.

- He completed one of the three tasks you asked him to do to get ready for bed. Tell him how great he did brushing his teeth and gently remind him of the two other things on the list.

- You didn't get a phone call from the school for the first time in a while. Don't dismiss it. Tell him how proud you are and how great he did that day!

As your child gets older, praise him for more specific victories. Don't continually praise for things that are so minute that it doesn't mean anything to him.

Sounds easy right? It is, but what if you can't see any positives? He's still failing in school, not paying attention, fighting with his siblings.

Then let me ask you this. Do you see any effort on his part? Probably so, because believe it or not, your child wants to please you.

He is not out to get you. His goal in life is not to make your life miserable!

He wants to do well, so my guess is, at least SOME of the time, he is putting forth effort.

If he's trying, that's an accomplishment. It's praiseworthy.

Give him an A for effort and praise him for it whenever you see it.

Key #2: ADD kids tend to be followers.

Note this! Inscribe this on your forehead!

It is imperative to instill self confidence in your child.

Follow the methods you learn in this book and watch his self-esteem skyrocket in just weeks.

It will work, but you have to work at it.

Your child may fail in many areas, get teased at school, and get in trouble a lot. When all of this is going on in his life, it can cause him to have strong feelings of inferiority. I can't tell you how many times I've had to try to "convince" Tena that she's smart. "I'm stupid" or "I'm just dumb like that" came out of her mouth way too many times.

You want your child to feel good about himself for the obvious reasons. You want him to be proud of himself, to feel like he can do well so that he will do well.

Children with low self esteem often fall into the wrong crowds. They lower their standards and end up where they feel they are more accepted and not judged. This can be the druggies, the promiscuous, the slouches, or the violent.

Again, I'm not trying to scare you but it's a minefield of delinquency out there and your kid will step on one if he feels badly enough about himself.

Confidence in oneself is important for so many reasons. Always affirm your child's strengths. Always let him know you are proud of specific accomplishments and always lift him up.

CHAPTER 3

Love, Forgiveness, and Respect

Please read carefully:

Love ... your ... child.

Wow. Again, telling you something you already know. Of course you love your child. Love is natural for a parent, the most basic parental instinct, a God-given gift.

Yes, I believe that's right.

However, sometimes love has to be a decision. Unfortunately we don't always feel the love, therefore it is not conveyed to our children.

Let's look at some things that might happen in your life, possibly on a daily basis.

- You get a call from the school – he's in trouble, again

- He didn't do what you asked – again

- He's late getting home or missed the bus – again

- He won't sit still and get his homework done – again

- He got a speeding ticket - again

Are you feeling the love?

I know you love him. But I also know he can zap you of all the patience and energy you have left. An ADD kid can suck the life right out of you until you're dangling at the very end of your rope.

I've been there, believe me. I have felt as though I didn't even like Tena, let alone love her, she had me so frustrated at times. It pains me even to say those words but it's the truth. There were times when the love wasn't anywhere to be found. It was buried deep in a dark place, under all the frustration, anger and hopelessness. It just couldn't find its way out.

Loving your child has to be a deliberate decision sometimes. Your basic love instinct can just fly out the window.

Think about it. He's in trouble again. He knows you're angry, exasperated. He knows he's messed up. He may even feel like he doesn't deserve to be loved. You don't like him right now.

But LOVE him anyway!

That sends an incredible, beautiful, powerful message that has immeasurable value. A message SO powerful it can transform a child.

You have got to understand the magnitude of this. This unconditional love can change everything.

Any time a child feels loved, it boosts his self-confidence, his self esteem, his self image. He feels valuable. That in itself is priceless.

But this is not the only benefit he will reap. This confidence and feeling of value gives him motivation to try harder, and to have the ability to do better, which ultimately results in greater success in his academic and social life. You cannot go wrong!

Be consistent. Always love him no matter what!

Let me give you an example of the power of love. Earlier I had mentioned Steven, a child I mentor in the public school. I go through a program called Kidshope, and it is geared for students considered "at risk". Kids that really need some one on one attention.

The success of this program is phenomenal! It has taken kids from academic failure to success, low self-confidence to high, social awkwardness to having friends and being accepted, aggressive behavior to non-aggressive - just to name a few of the amazing changes this program has seen. And it's attributed to the love and attention they get from someone who was once a stranger.

How much more can be accomplished with your own child, since you can spend much more than once a week encouraging him, spending quality time with him, talking with him and accepting him the way he is.

Now having said that...

When your child needs correction, when he gets in trouble, loving him does NOT mean that you can't get angry. It doesn't mean there shouldn't be consequences. Just be sure to administer consequences in love, not in anger. Walk away if you are feeling too angry to deal with him reasonably. Too often we parents can say things we should not say in our anger. Once the words are out, they can't be taken back. They can do severe damage.

You will get angry, and rightly so.

But always love in the end.

Now on to forgiveness.

You can't just love your child; you have to forgive him. Say it and mean it. Forgiveness frees both of you. It will relieve him of the feeling of being a disappointment or feeling he will never measure up. It will free you of the negative energy that builds up when you hold on to things, causing tension and a lack of peace.

You are the adult. Don't hold grudges, don't give the silent treatment. Model forgiveness for your child, and give him the grace he deserves.

This goes both ways. Your child is not the only one who needs forgiveness. You will also need it. There will be times (many in fact) that you need this from your child. Fortunately, kids are generally very forgiving!

There were times I got so angry with Tena that I was hurtful and unfair. I thought she could never forgive me. I was even afraid to ask sometimes. But she always did, completely and wholly.

But be sure and ask. Show that respect and humility. It speaks volumes!

And don't forget...

Forgive yourself!

You are human, and you react in human ways. Any kid can bring out the worst in a parent, but a kid with ADD can do it even more so. Know that you will make mistakes, but every day is a new day. Don't beat yourself up. Forgive yourself and go on.

Lastly, the next powerful little word ... Respect.

Please respect your child!

Wait! Hold on. He needs to respect me ... I'm the parent. Yes, absolutely. He needs to respect you.

But you must also respect your child.

R-E-S-P-E-C-T ... find out what it means to me.

Remember this old Aretha Franklin song?

Ok, I'm dating myself. Maybe this is before your time.

But there is wisdom in this short lyric. When you respect your child, you'll find out exactly what it means to him.

A little respect will do wonders for his self-confidence. It can make the difference between night and day.

How does one do this?

Quite simply, demonstrate to your child that you value his opinion, and that you believe that his opinion and ideas are worthwhile.

My friend Megan is a great example of this concept. Tyler is ADHD (with the H.) Megan and her husband pulled Tyler out of public school in the middle of 6th grade, and Megan began homeschooling him. Tyler initially had a lot of trouble focusing at home especially when he did lessons online. Instead of doing his lesson, he would often gravitate to YouTube or some other social media website.

Megan tried everything to get him to stay on task, but only one thing worked. She started to ask him what was causing him to be distracted.

Is the work too hard, do you feel you need a break, how can I help? Oftentimes Tyler was able to verbalize whatever it was that he needed or what he thought might help him concentrate.

Not only did this solve the problem of getting his work done, but Tyler felt respected by his mom. SHE asked HIM! She needed his help! His opinion, advice, and ideas were valuable.

The change in demeanor she saw in him when she started to do this was nothing short of amazing. He was more confident and more motivated to do well. He actually started staying on task.

Key #3: Let your child be in control!

Yikes! Most people don't like that one.

Let me soften this for you a bit by explaining exactly what I mean.

When you show your child respect by asking for his help, the way Megan did with Tyler, it gives him a sense of control.

Kids with ADD often feel out of control. They can't help a lot of the things they do. They get out of their seat, blurt out, zone out. They don't want to do these things but they happen, and then they get reprimanded for it.

When you ask him for help, get his opinion, implement his ideas, it helps him feel valuable but also in control.

Let's look at another common scenario and see how a parent can handle showing respect and giving some control over to the child.

So once again, he is running late and misses the school bus.

Parent: Why do you think you're late to the bus a lot?

GIVE HIM A FEW MINUTES TO THINK ABOUT IT.

Child: I don't know (or deafening silence).

Parent: Why don't you think about it? Think through your morning and see if you can figure out what might hold you up.

The next day, remind him to follow his list of what to do in the morning and to pay attention to what he actually does. You pay attention as well.

One of you may notice that he had to look for his shoes for 5 minutes or that he plays with his breakfast. If he noticed something on his own, that's fantastic. If not, you can tell him what you noticed and ask him what he thinks can be done to remedy it.

Parent: I noticed you couldn't find your shoes. Do you think that might cause you to run a little behind? OR

Parent: I noticed you played with your breakfast and it took you a while to eat. Do you think that's why you might miss the bus sometimes?

If he agrees, ask him how he thinks he can fix the problem. Why he plays with his breakfast. Ask him, "is it because you don't like it? "What would you rather eat?"

"How can we fix the problem of having to look for your shoes?"

Of course, the ability for your child to think through these things, to notice the problem and come up with solutions, will largely depend on his age and maturity. If he is 5 years old, you may need to tell him what you see as the problem and possible solutions. But even if you have to do that, ask his opinion.

Example:

Parent: I noticed you playing with your food. Don't you like your breakfast?

Child: Not really.

Parent: Do you think it takes longer for you to eat when you have oatmeal because you don't like it that much?

Child: I guess.

Parent: What would you rather eat for breakfast?

Child: I don't know

Parent: I know you like waffles. Would you like waffles in the mornings?

Child: I guess.

Parent: Do you think if you had waffles you wouldn't play with your food as much and would get finished with breakfast faster?

Child: Maybe

Parent: Why don't we try that tomorrow? That's a great idea you had to have waffles next time.

Give him credit for thinking up the solution even though in reality you came up with it. Not only does this help him feel respected and in control, it helps him learn to problem solve on his own!

This can be life changing for a child. Let me reiterate what I said in summary about love, because the same goes for respect.

Any time a child feels respected, it boosts his self-confidence, his self esteem, his self image. He feels valuable. That in itself is priceless.

But this is not the only benefit he will reap. This confidence and feeling of value gives him motivation to try harder, and to have the ability to do better, which ultimately results in greater success in his academic and social life. You cannot go wrong!

If you learn nothing else from this book, please take to heart and implement what you've learned about love, respect and belief from this chapter. The power packed in these three little concepts is the greatest secret to your child's success!

Chapter 4

Easy - but Powerful – Strategies

This is probably one of the topics you've been waiting for: to find out what you can actually DO. Enough of all this mind and thinking stuff you say. I want some practical, useful information!

Ok, here it comes. But let me remind you, everything you have read so far is imperative!

You can use all the greatest strategies in the world with your child, but without the right mindset, the love, respect and forgiveness, it will all be for naught. Remember that, and as you use the strategies presented to you, use them in conjunction with the right frame of mind.

First, I will provide a list of some practical, easy but amazingly effective strategies you can use beginning immediately. I will elaborate on some of them later in this chapter.

Keep this list in a safe but easily accessible place. Laminate it. Use it every day!

You ready?

1. Maintain eye contact with your child when giving instructions or directions. This will help him to focus on what you are saying.

2. Have him repeat directions/instructions back to you.

3. Teach him to sit closer to the edge of his chair and lean forward when trying to listen.

4. Use immediate rewards. ADD children generally do not have a good concept of "future."

5. Limit his time with media like video games and television. Children get used to the overstimulation and entertainment and find it harder to focus on something like a history lesson.

6. Read TO your child from a very young age, until he won't let you read to him anymore.

7. Be sure he gets some free outdoor play time every day.

8. Keep your child in a routine. Keep him to a schedule as much as possible. Specific ideas for this are in the next chapter on structure.

9. When changing the child's activity - for example - having him come from playing outside to coming inside for dinner, give him time to adjust to the change in activity.

10. Use checklists, alarm clocks, all the tools you can think of to keep him organized and focused. Specific ideas for this are in the next chapter on structure.

11. Incorporate some quiet time into his day, where he plays a game or reads a book for example (if he likes to read of course.)

12. Spend time each evening reviewing the next day's events.

13. When explaining or giving directions, keep it short.

14. Teach him to count to 5 before speaking. This will help inhibit the inappropriate speaking out of turn.

15. Try to get him to journal a little each day. When journaling regularly, one begins to get thoughts, worries and frustrations on paper. This practice can be very therapeutic and useful for balancing mood and reducing anxiety.

Some of these could use a little more explanation, so allow me to elaborate:

First, I'll address using immediate rewards. ADD children generally do not have a good concept of the future. The fact that doing something now (like studying hard) will benefit him later, just does not compute.

He doesn't think that far ahead. Studying is just another thing he has to do for which he sees no benefit. So you need to reward him in smaller intervals. If he studies for a test very diligently one day, praise him and reward him. Give him a break from one of his chores or extra time doing an activity he enjoys. It is important to reward your child for small steps.

The timing of how often you reward and for what behaviors you reward will depend on the age and maturity of your child and on past experience. You will have to be the judge of that. Just remember that no matter what the age, the future is somewhere on another planet for your ADD kid. It's nowhere to be seen.

Next, read to your child! This is of utmost importance!

This is one of the things I could kick myself for. I did not do this long enough with Tena. I read to her till she was about eight and when I did read, I didn't read regularly enough. I believe that is one of the reasons she hates to read and why her reading comprehension, vocabulary and critical thinking skills are still not up to par.

Reading has intellectual, social, and behavioral implications. The benefits are astounding.

- Numerous studies have shown that students who are exposed to reading before preschool have a higher aptitude for learning.

- Reading is essential for all aspects of life. It's necessary for learning other subjects in school, to fill out applications, for jobs, reading contracts, and just for life in general! Knowing how to read and comprehend is imperative!

- Being read to (and reading on one's own) teaches your child thinking skills. He learns cause and effect, how to exercise logic, and how to think abstractly.

- He learns the formation of language and sounds.

- He learns to stay focused. He will develop stronger self-discipline and a longer attention span.

- Reading aids in memory retention.

- He will learn to love to read. Often kids who love to read will choose reading a book over video games or other less productive forms of entertainment.

- Reading helps improve vocabulary.

- Reading improves writing ability.

Sometimes hearing helps your child to comprehend better. Audiobooks are a fantastic tool. Many are available at your local library and online.

I have a nephew who is a reading maniac. Almost every time I see him he has his nose in a book. I remember one Christmas when he was about 10 years old and our family was all together (about 40 of us), and Max was sitting on the couch reading a book. His cousins were playing and screaming, food was being passed around, and excitement was in the air. Max didn't seem to notice. He could focus on that book like a laser beam. He loves to read, and he has already benefitted greatly from it.

There's even more benefits than I have listed here. Please do not underestimate the power of the written word.

Next:

Be sure he gets some free outdoor play time every day.

Whether your child is the hyperactive type, inattentive or combined, outdoor play time is a major benefit. Outdoor play stimulates creative thought processes. It's also been known to build self-confidence in children and can relieve stress.

Help him by giving him time to do something fun, to be outside, get some fresh air and exercise. It can do wonders!

When changing the child's activity - for example, having him come inside for dinner - give him time to adjust to the change from outdoor play to sitting at the dinner table.

ADD children often have trouble shifting from one activity to the next. When ADD kids are involved in an activity, it requires shift in mindset to change it and it takes some time. If your child is playing outside, for example, and it's time to come in for dinner, it will be very difficult for him to stop what he's doing, come in and sit down at the dinner table. That's hard for most kids but even harder for the kid with ADD.

Don't just call him in and expect him to settle down and you all have a nice quiet family dinner!

Make sure he knows how much time he has to play outside, what time he needs to come in. Call him or have him set his watch for 5 or 10 minutes before that time. Tell him when he has just 1 or 2 more minutes. When he comes in, let him wash up and take a few minutes to calm down and settle in before he sits at the table.

Even switching from one subject to another while doing homework can be a problem for him. He may NEED the change, but then he can't start focusing on a new subject or task when he's been involved in another one. Be patient and just remember that you need to give him time to mentally shift from one thing to another. Just giving a warning a couple of minutes beforehand can make all the difference.

When explaining or giving directions, keep it short.

When talking to Tena, either explaining directions or just trying to make a point, I would tend go on and on ... and on, repeating myself, rewording, elaborating. After all, she needed more explanation, more detail. She's ADD.

NO!

The more you talk the more you lose them. I continued this way for years until one day Tena said, "Mom, I lost you way back at (blank)." It was then that I realized that the more I talked, the more I lost or confused her.

Be short and concise. Then ask him if he has any questions. At that point you can resume talking! Know that the longer you go, the less he hears.

Give these strategies a try. Be consistent with them. I think you will be amazed at the results you see.

Ok, time for another key ingredient.

Key #4: Lower your expectations.

What!

Yes, you heard me right.

There may be dozens of things in your child that need improvement to help him succeed in life. But there is only so much he can handle at once.

Don't try to teach him homework strategies, social skills and how to keep his room organized all at the same time. Focus on one or two things.

Choose what you think is the most detrimental to his well-being, or that may be dangerous to him or others. Those things need to be addressed first. As an illustration:

He's failing math class.

He has a fit almost every time you take him out somewhere.

He doesn't do his chores.

Maybe these are the three top concerns with him right now. In addition, he is extremely disorganized, and very easily frustrated.

Choose one, at the most two, to focus on right now. Decide which is most important.

Choose and then work hard at it. If it's the grades you decide on, work with him on strategies to help with his schoolwork. Give positive reinforcement and rewards along the way. Make sure you have variety in the rewards to keep him interested.

When you see him begin to master the behavior, wean him off of the rewards then tackle the next behavior.

Do not try to fix everything at once. Take one step at a time.

Basically, just keep your expectations reasonable. Any child can be overwhelmed with too much at once, especially the ADD child!

Strategies for a Meltdown

This is a biggie. Meltdown and tantrums are much more prevalent in the life of the ADD child.

Sometimes things can get way out of hand. Children with ADD can be very sensitive to stimulation. Places with bright lights, lots of activity, noise, crowds - these can over stimulate your child to a point where he becomes highly agitated. Frustration can mount to the point of anger and into a meltdown or temper tantrum. If you have gone through this with your child, you know how frustrating and embarrassing it can be.

You're at the grocery store. He wants a candy bar. He asks, you answer no.

He asks again, and again.

You don't let him have one and he starts having a fit. He may be 10 years old. He looks like any other "normal" child out there.

Then it starts ... the dreaded tantrum. And with it, the stares, the shaking heads and the looks that say, "can't she control her kid?" "What is wrong with him? What kind of parent is she?"

You want to crawl under a rock.

It's ok. It happens to the best of us. But there are ways to handle these outbursts effectively or avoid them altogether.

Get out your highlighter and let's go through this together.

First, be a boy scout - Be prepared! Before you go on one of these outings, prepare him for it.

You probably know your child's triggers. If you don't, you will soon - I guarantee it.

Try to prevent this in the first place. I'll use the example of an outing to the grocery store.

Talk with him before you go. Let him know where you're going and what you expect from him. If you know he'll want candy and you don't want him to have it, tell him you're not buying candy this time.

Plan ahead for a reward he will get at home for his good behavior. Remind him periodically, while you are out, of your conversation about your expectations and of the reward awaiting him.

Keep him busy. Holding something or playing with something can help. Try a stress ball, silly putty or give him a pencil with a pad of paper to draw on.

Depending on his age, you might let him help you scratch items off your list as you pick them up, or have him help you pick out items from the shelf. If he's old enough, have him tell you what the prices are on items you're about to put in your cart.

Play some kind of game with him while you're shopping. Try an I-Spy game, for example. He'll be focused on searching for something and may not even notice all that's going on around him.

Do these kinds of things consistently - every time you go out.

Now, I hate to say it, but it's true. Unfortunately, despite your efforts, your child may not be able to help himself if he is truly too sensitive to the environment you are in.

If this is the case, make your trips short or avoid taking him with you if possible. Leave him home with dad or older sibling or a trusted neighbor. Try again at a later time.

Ok, sounds good, Karen, but what if I have no choice? He has to go with me.

Take these simple steps.

Once it starts, make yourself eye level with your child. This conveys a sense that you are with him, not against him.

Talk to him in a quiet and controlled voice. Do not exacerbate the situation by screaming back at him.

Watch your tone of voice. Do not speak with an angry or condescending tone.

If it continues, you may need to find a restroom to hide out in until he calms down. You may need to go outside or just go home. Leaving is not a sign of defeat. It's just a necessity sometimes. Don't let it get you down. Try again when you think you are both ready.

Key #5: Teach Don't Punish

Note! Punishing can backfire!

Be careful about how you discipline your child.

I know - I've done it plenty of times. "Tena, you didn't clean up your toys. Go to your room." "Tena, that was disrespectful! Write "I will be respectful" 50 times."

If you'll remember from a previous chapter, often these kids are just acting out negative feelings. They are not trying to be disruptive or "bad."

When you punish him for behavior he cannot control, the ramifications are detrimental to both of you. He will feel resentment toward you. He will feel more out of control than usual, he'll feel defeated. It will add to his already compromised self-confidence and self-esteem. If he can't control the behavior, consequences can backfire big time.

So what do I do? Just let it go?

No.

But the best teacher is the law of nature. You touch the stove, you get burned.

What you do is allow or administer "natural" consequences for negative behavior.

Understand this however! I am not saying let him touch the stove so he'll get burned and he'll learn never to do that again. By all means, stop him and let him know what will happen if he touches it!

There are actually ways to teach him without using "punishment." You use the natural consequence of a behavior instead. This teaches him what happens when he does this and what happens when he doesn't do that.

Let me give you some real life examples.

John is dilly dallying around at homework time and doesn't get his homework done. You have set the timer; all strategies are in place to help him stay on task. But he just doesn't do it.

Normally maybe he gets to watch TV for 30 minutes after his homework is finished.

The natural consequence would be that he doesn't get to do that. He has to finish his homework and probably have to forgo that free time. It's probably not necessary, nor would it be effective, to send him to his room or to make him write "I will do my homework" on a sheet of paper 50 times! It teaches him nothing.

When you allow the natural consequence of missing TV, he sees that this is a direct result of him not doing what he was supposed to do. It's a great life lesson that he will carry into adulthood:

He doesn't get his resume done; he doesn't get a job; he doesn't finish the project; his boss reprimands or fires him. He needs to learn these lessons, and life is the best teacher.

If you'll remember, my friend Megan pulled her son Tyler out of school to homeschool him. He had some of his classes online. This posed a problem. When he was on the computer, he was always browsing on You Tube and Facebook instead of doing his work!

He did better when she let him help her think of solutions. He did still get distracted sometimes, however, so he got behind in his work. The natural consequence his mom allowed was that he had to work on weekends and over Christmas break to catch up. You get behind then you work on your free time. He caught on pretty quick!

These examples are naturally occurring consequences. You just have to allow them to happen. Don't feel bad that little Johnny doesn't get to watch TV. He didn't finish his homework so he doesn't. You might need to sit down with him and help him get through his homework and let him take the breaks he needs, but TV doesn't happen!

Let me give you an example of what I mean by "administering natural consequences."

This happened one day when Tena was about 4 years old and we went to the grocery store. On the way home I noticed there was a bag of chips in one of my grocery bags that I did not remember buying! I asked her about it and she said she saw them on our way out and put them in one of our grocery bags. She had no idea she was stealing. She just saw it, wanted it, and grabbed it.

Well, tempting as it was to continue on and enjoy my free bag of chips, I gently explained to Tena that it belongs to the store, and we can't just take it, we have to pay for it. When you don't pay it's called stealing and it's against the law and morally wrong. I told her we were taking it back, and she would have to apologize to the cashier. She didn't want to do it, and she was scared, but she did it.

I believe it's natural that when you commit a wrongdoing against someone, you should apologize for it. The cashier nearly fell over when Tena confessed and returned the chips. She thanked Tena and was happy to see this little girl doing the right thing! Tena felt good about it and learned a valuable lesson.

So do your best to take advantage of every teachable moment. When your child sees the natural ramifications of a behavior over and over again, he'll learn - and he will be all the better for it.

Sometimes, however, there may not be a "natural consequence" of a behavior and you feel you must deliver some other kind of discipline or punishment. By all means, use your best judgment.

You are the parent, and you know your child best.

Also --- I'm sure I don't have to tell you, but I will anyway. If he is engaging in something dangerous to himself or others, do what you have to do.

If he is running in the street after you've told him three times to come back in the yard, don't wait till he gets hit by a car! That is not the kind of natural consequences I 'm talking about. For goodness sake, grab him, bring him in and make him sit in time out or write "I will not play in the street" 50 times if you have to. If there's not a reasonable natural consequence, teach him the best way you can.

I know the strategies in this chapter work. Some will work better for your child than others, but I encourage you to try what you're comfortable with and then... be consistent, and persistent.

Don't be kicking yourself 10 years from now for not learning or implementing things that may have really benefitted your child.

You have one shot at life. Make it count!

CHAPTER 5

Structures and Schedules

You see it every day. He's running late; he doesn't know where his homework is; he can't decide what to wear. He's all over the place.

ADD kids need an external system to help them get and stay organized. They don't have the built in mechanisms to do it themselves. They need structure!

I remember during Tena's middle school years she would often come home from school upset because she felt she had failed a test. When I ask her why, I would hear this proclamation, "I didn't know we were having a test! The teacher never said anything!"

This is when I implemented the Keep An Agenda idea. It should have been implemented much earlier but I was always such a micromanager she didn't really need one. I do not recommend micromanaging by the way. Teaching them to do things themselves works much better!

We picked an agenda from the local Target and she learned to write everything down. Little by little, tests became less of a surprise.

Today's technology can be extremely useful for kids with ADD. To tell you the truth, I resist the modern electronics. I HATE cell phones and honestly wish they had never been invented.

I believe they have changed communication in a way that is detrimental to building and strengthening relationships - they have made it almost impossible for parents to be in their kids' business the way they should! I hate to hear my kids pick up their cell and start talking with I-have-no-idea-whom. I long for the land line to ring, pick it up and talk first with whomever is calling my daughter.

But I digress. It is what it is.

Honestly though, the I-phones and smart phones are a blessing in some ways for the ADD kid. I have a love-hate relationship with them, but sometimes I think if the I-phone could walk, I'd kiss the ground it walked on. There's the love part of my love-hate.

It is amazingly easy to keep track of any number of things with these phones.

Your child can keep his agenda in there. He can set it up to give himself reminders. He can have instant access to a calculator and a dictionary. He can jot down notes to himself.

It can help him stay on schedule. For example, he could set his phone to ring at 4:30 pm every day to remind him to start his homework. He can set a reminder for 6:00 pm to be at the dinner table...whatever he needs. If his phone has Siri on it, a talking "personal assistant", he can even receive verbal reminders. This can be an ideal tool for the ADD child.

If he's not that tech savvy, he's too young, or he doesn't have a phone, no problem. An agenda or some type of calendar is perfect.

When used consistently, your child will eventually learn to take control of his time and his schedule, and many of these daily living responsibilities will become second nature.

Key #6: Structure is necessary and liberating, not boring and tedious.

It can be simple for your child to maintain a schedule - an agenda, a phone, charts! It doesn't take a lot of work but it does work.

Checklists and Charts

Not boring and tedious! These can actually be fun!

Checklists and charts are a sadly under-used but extremely powerful tool in helping your child to get and stay on track.

They take the pressure off of him to remember and it takes the pressure off of you to endlessly remind him.

Below is an example of a chart for an after school schedule.

TIME	TASK	PICTURE	M	T	W	TH	F
3:45	Clean out backpack						
4:00	Watch TV or play video games						
4:30	Snack time						
4:45	Home-work						

Depending on his age, your child may not need or want the picture. But for young children it is extremely helpful.

Be more specific if you need to: for example have starting and ending times or write in what snack for each day.

Attach privileges or rewards to the number of checkmarks each day or each week. This will help him to be vigilant about looking at it, doing what it says, and marking it when he's done. Eventually, he'll get it and the external rewards can go away.

A chart is an easy and wondrously useful tool. Laminate them and use dry erase markers. You can have these things up for as long as you need them!

You can use a chart like this for chores, for bedtime routines, for early morning routines, anything your heart desires.

Speaking of routines, I cannot stress their importance enough! Your child needs to know what is happening when, and what he needs to do when. Sometimes plans change, and it can't be helped, but stick to a regular schedule and routine as much as possible.

He Never Reached the Finish Line!

What if your child gets started on something, at exactly the time he was scheduled to do so, but he just doesn't finish it?

In the middle of cleaning his room, he gets a text and next thing you know, the time has gone, and he's managed to hang one shirt and that's it.

Your first reaction when you see his room might be to get angry and tell him he didn't do what you asked, then tell him to do it now ... or else.

Or you might give him 15 more minutes and say it better be done when you get back.

Or maybe you'll fly off the handle and ground him for the next 3 weeks.

Let me give you an alternative strategy. Kids need structure, right? Sometimes having too much unsupervised time to complete a task does not work. He is too easily distracted.

Try smaller increments of time. First find something to praise him for. Always praise if you can! If he did something, notice it and acknowledge it.

Tell him something like, "I see you put some shirts away. That's great. But now I need you to put away the rest of your clothes. I'll be back in 5 minutes to see how you're doing."

Come back in 5 minutes. Hopefully, he got more clothes put away. Compliment him on what he's done, give him another 5 minutes to get the rest of the clothes picked up. This could go on five times longer than you anticipated but in the end the job will be done.

Your child will have accomplished what he set out to do, and you don't have to look at this train wreck of a room any longer!

Telling an ADD child to just "go clean your room," or "clean up the kitchen," is not always enough.

Often your child needs explicit step by step instruction:

- Hang up your shirts.

- Make the bed.

- Put dirty clothes in the hamper.

- Put trash in the waste basket.

- Straighten up your dresser.

You may have to write it down. Eventually he'll do it on his own.

I can't count the number of times I've told Tena to do something without thinking how involved the task really was. The idea of cleaning your room, to me, is simple. Just go clean it.

But there's so much more to it. It means hang things, straighten things, throw things away. Every small task can be overwhelming for our children with ADD.

Location, Location, Location

Your child also needs his things to be organized. Everything he uses should be stored in the same place. Clothes, toys, books, school supplies, sports equipment. He needs to know exactly where things are located so he can find them easily and without frustration.

Use bins, baskets, shelves, boxes. These are invaluable tools! Start with your child's room. Books on one shelf, toys in one or two baskets, underwear and socks in one drawer, shorts in another, shirts in another. Label the drawers and shelves.

It is a great idea to have your child do the organizing with you. He will remember more clearly where things are because he helped decide to put them there and he is physically placing things where they go. It also gives him a sense of control and accomplishment.

The Morning Rush

"Where's my backpack?" Where's my homework?" "I don't know what to eat for breakfast!"

Mornings can be hazardous to your health. You're late again. He can't find anything, he can't make a decision. You're about to lose your mind!

Remember my admonition to you when you are getting ready to go out somewhere?

Be a Boy Scout. Be prepared!

Each night before bed, follow these simple steps. You may have to help him or do it for him if he's a younger child.

He should have his clothes picked out and ready to wear for the next day.

He should decide what he will eat for breakfast and have it out on the counter or have it ready to take out of the fridge.

He should put everything he needs for school in his backpack.

His backpack should be by the door.

If he brings lunch to school, the lunch should be in there or if it needs to be refrigerated, then a note on top of the backpack that says, "GET LUNCH."

His shoes should be next to his backpack.

In the morning, if he has a morning routine chart, remind him to look at it and check things off.

Easy and well worth it! Your mornings will be so much more peaceful. You will not believe the difference this will make for him AND for you!

Make this part of your regular routine.

At the end of the day, bedtime routine should always be the same. You might have a chart for it. Brush teeth, wash face, set alarm.

Before he goes to sleep, it's a fantastic idea to spend a little time with your child. After he crawls into bed use this time to read to him and/or just to talk. Talk about whatever comes to his mind or ask him questions about his day. Many children will open up to you at this time. It's a great opportunity for bonding, for your child to confide in you, and for you to get a glimpse into some of his worries or fears.

Tena would always do most of her talking at night before bed. Maybe it was a stall tactic, I don't know! It really doesn't matter. I learned a lot about her during those little talks. I learned about things that happened at school, good or bad, I learned if she was worried or angry about something, if she was excited or happy. It was a time for her to get things off her chest and for me to help her work through them. The time was priceless.

Routine helps calm your child because he knows what will happen next. The schedule alleviates confusion, helps him stay on task and helps him feel in control.

Structure, routine, schedule.

Such simple things with so much benefit.

Chapter 6

School - Can We Just Skip These 12 Years?

Key #7: Teachers and administrators don't always do what's best for your kid.

Shocking? Maybe, maybe not.

How is the school situation working out for you?

I am literally shocked by some of the stories I hear and read about in regards to how children with ADD are treated in the schools. I am shocked by how the parents of these children are treated.

It can seriously be a nightmare.

Teachers who should be well-trained in the area of special needs and ADHD often seem to know nothing about it. Teachers, who you would expect to be compassionate, patient, and persistent in working with you and your child, sometimes seem like they couldn't care less. It's like your kid is an inconvenience, a burden.

Allow me to digress for one moment: As a side note, I know this is not every teacher. I am sorry if I have offended anyone out there. Your child's teacher may be awesome, or you may even be a teacher yourself (if you are, I'm sure you're an awesome one as well.) I know there are incredible teachers out there. Tena had a lot of them.

But, as many of you parents have seen or experienced, there are those teachers who just don't seem to care or understand your plight and the plight of your child. Teachers who don't seem to know anything about ADD or are just plain rude and condescending.

Some administrative bodies are no better. They take literally months to look over your child's psychological evaluations or to test them at school, then to finally meet with you and then at long last... get them into the appropriate programs. They don't talk with the uncooperative teacher for you; they don't meet with you when you need to talk with them.

I had my own challenges with finding a good fit for Tena. That is why I moved this poor little thing from school to school for her entire school career.

She started in full time private school and from there, I tried solely homeschooling. After that, a hybrid school (two days in school, three days at home), then to a different hybrid, then to public school, then back to yet another hybrid for her 10th grade year through graduation. Whew! My poor guinea pig.

Most of the teachers Tena had were fantastic. The administrators were great. However, most weren't able to adjust their methods enough to really help her, hard as they tried.

And I didn't know enough to be much help to them either.

Tena managed to get decent grades, but guess what she didn't get?

An education!

Can any of you relate to that? How can you get good grades if you haven't really learned? Is your child getting an education?

The education system failed. Tena passed every grade with mostly A's and B's, but she didn't learn much. Finally, in 10th grade, I made that one last school move. It worked out beautifully. Unfortunately we didn't find the right fit for her until her sophomore year in high school. I wish it had been sooner but as the saying goes: "better late than never."

So trust me when I say that I know school can be a challenge. Finding the right fit can be difficult if not impossible.

I was lucky though. For the most part the teachers and administrators cared and they really tried. This is not always the case.

As you may recall from a previous chapter, I told you a story about my friend Megan and her son Tyler, who has ADHD.

Tyler is classic ADHD, and it had a profound effect on his school experience.

Megan noticed it when he was in 3rd grade.

- Tyler didn't understand a lot of the material, and his reading level was low.

- If a kid behind him was tapping his pencil, Tyler lost all focus.

- He missed information and missed or misunderstood directions.

- He would "blurt out" things in the middle of class. For example, if he saw a hair on his desk he would blurt out, "there's a hair on my desk!"

- He got out of his seat.

- He goofed off.

Of course, Tyler was reprimanded every time. After too many infractions of one kind or another, he would be sent to the principal's office. Then that would morph into detention for having too many trips to the principal's office.

The more the teachers put their thumb on him, the more he pushed back.

Things got so bad that Tyler started to hate school, and he thought one of his teachers hated him.

He started having stomach aches in the morning and couldn't eat.

A vicious cycle in the classroom began. When Tyler would goof off, or blurt things out, kids would think it was funny. This gave Tyler a feeling of belonging, so he would start to intentionally do it more. Kids even started asking him to randomly ask things of the teacher in the middle of class just to see him do it and watch him get in trouble.

He gained a reputation with the teachers and staff as a troublemaker. When he was with a group of kids and they were all being rambunctious, he was the one who was singled out and corrected or punished.

In his 3rd grade year, Tyler had a fabulous teacher who tried to work with him but she enabled him more than helped him. He passed with flying colors but did not earn the grades he got.

Tyler's 4th grade teacher did not cooperate with his parents at all. She called him out and embarrassed him in front of the class. When Megan and her husband approached her with strategies they wanted her to try with him, her response was, "No, I don't do it that way."

His fifth grade teacher had an autistic son and understood learning differences and behavioral disorders. She took a different approach with Tyler. She would reward good behavior and break assignments up for him. She did not call Tyler out but would subtly correct him so as not to embarrass him in front of his peers.

And so the roller coaster went. Good teachers, caring teachers, not so caring teachers.

The last straw came when Tyler was in the 7th grade. One of his teachers seemed to have it out for him. She constantly blamed him for things he didn't do. She only tried a recommended strategy once for him, breaking a test up into smaller bits (chunking as Tyler called it). When she did this, Tyler did significantly better, and she saw the improvement. But she never did it again. She was rude and impatient with him.

In November of that year, Tyler and his parents met with the teacher for a conference. They asked her why she thought Tyler wasn't improving and how she was working with him in the classroom. Her response was, "This is a world class school. Tyler is lucky to be here." Very defensive.

When Megan asked her why she did not continue to break tests up for Tyler when it was obvious that it had helped him before, her response was (and she addressed Tyler) "You really like to hold on to that chunking thing, don't you?"

When she saw that she upset him, and he was on the verge of tears, she said to him, very condescendingly, "I know it's hard Tyler, it's really hard."

At that point, Tyler's dad got up, announced "we're done," and they all walked out, never to darken the doors of that school again.

After that, mid-November of Tyler's 7th grade year, Megan started an online homeschooling program with him.

This lack of empathy, cooperation and stunning lack of compassion this family experienced is mind-boggling. I hope you never have to go through anything like this with your child. But unfortunately this is a reality for many people.

So what do you do?

Take matters into your own hands. You have to be super involved in your child's education. It's hard, especially if you have other kids, a job, or other things sapping you of time and energy.

I don't want the stories of Tena and Tyler to scare you. It doesn't mean that school will not work out for your child. Every person, every school is different.

But you have to remember this: you care about your child, and you may be the only one who cares when it comes to his education.

Be involved! Make a pest of yourself. Don't let up.

Your child needs an advocate. Keep tabs on his learning, check his grades online, help him with his homework. Help him study for tests, quiz him, work with him. Make sure he is learning.

Work with the school and don't give up!

- Be persistent,

- Meet regularly with the teacher(s), principal, guidance counselor.

- Go as high up on the ladder as you need to go for help.

- Write to the superintendent of the school district if you have to.

- Make them put your child's needs first!

The thing is, even though teachers and the administration may be trained or educated in how to work with ADD children, they don't seem to get it sometimes. So here's what you do:

You Educate Them!

Yes, educate the educated.

Explain what your child's weaknesses and traits are. Explain what ADD is (in a way that won't make them feel like you think they're an idiot, if possible!) and tell them you want to work together to figure out ways to help your child succeed in school.

If your child has an IEP (Individual Education Plan) or an EIP (Early Intervention Program), you probably were present for the planning of strategies put on that plan. Make sure those are being implemented. If you don't think that what is on there is sufficient, tell the teacher that you have other things you believe will help and ask him or her to work with you to implement these new ideas.

Below are some ideas that can help your child in the school setting. Some of these should be easy for the teacher to integrate into the class. Some are not so easy but they can be done.

Don't be intimidated by the length of this list! Read through it; take from it what makes sense to you. If they all make sense, know you do NOT have to approach the teacher with all of them right away. Talk to her about what you think would be most beneficial to your child first, then add some in as the weeks and months go by.

NOTE: Many of these strategies can be used at home as well. When used consistently at home and school, the benefits will be tenfold.

Ask the teacher to try some of these ideas and strategies:

- Seat your child in the front row and make frequent eye contact with him. Also tap him on the shoulder or tap his desk to get his attention when he seems distracted or is zoning out. Small movements like this can help him concentrate better, and they won't distract the other students.

- Use his name often. This will aid in redirecting him back to the lesson.

- Never call on him when he appears to be in another world. This is embarrassing for him, and he doesn't have control over it.

- Allow him to leave the room when he is too fidgety or restless.

- He can have a signal to let the teacher know he needs to leave the room, or the teacher can even have pre-written notes saying, "Ben needs to take a walk," for example. He will give the note to the teacher; he will walk to the office; and they will know to send a note back with him so other students think he was just running an errand.

- Allow him to have a snack if he feels he is losing concentration and needs some brain fuel. The teacher may need to allow the rest of the class this same privilege, which I personally think is a good practice. All kids need some fuel for the brain throughout the day.

- Check his agenda or planner at the end of the day or at the end of each class to make sure he wrote down all homework assignments and upcoming tests. Or have a responsible friend you all agree on who will compare notes with your child and make sure he wrote everything down.

- Allow him to use colored paper to write on. This can often help with focusing.

- Allow him to chew gum or listen to an ipod while doing class work. Contrary to popular belief, multi-tasking can help some kids, especially those with ADD, to focus better on a task.

- Let him help with things like cleaning the board, stacking chairs, gathering balls from the playground. This helps with the restlessness and excess energy. He will get it out in productive ways, and it will also help him feel useful and important!

- Never discipline him by having him lose recess or PE or any other activity that is a good outlet for his excess energy.

- Ask him periodically if what you (teacher) are doing is helping him or not. Ask if he has any other ideas or suggestions that will help him to understand better or help him pay attention more.

- If he is good in a certain subject(s) ask him to help other students. This is a win-win for your child, the other student, and the teacher.

- Give consistent positive reinforcement for any good behavior and also for a decrease in poor behavior.

- Have the class start with a little exercise ... jumping jacks, running in place. Also have breaks like this during class. This is good for all the kids. It helps get the brain and body stimulated, release excess energy, and remove boredom.

- When explaining assignments, break the instructions into steps, or divide a project into categories and let your child work on one at a time.

- Keep a colored post it on his desk. When he exhibits good behavior/proper control, etc. during class, the teacher can periodically mark it with checkmarks. When he reaches a certain number of checkmarks, he receives a privilege or reward decided upon beforehand.

- Change activity every 15 minutes. Sometimes changes will have to be subtle so they are not noticeable to other students (such as moving from answering questions to reading)

- Let him use a ruler or colored paper to scan down while he reads to help him keep his place and reduce the anxiety caused by seeing too much text at once.

- Stay in regular communication with you. Work with you in deciding what to continue, change, or alter depending on how well thing seem to be working.

Some of these will work better than others for your child. Ask the teacher to try what YOU think will be beneficial. Get her input and see what she thinks. Keep what works, throw out what doesn't.

What an astounding difference this will make in your child! And what a difference it will make in the entire class if she implements some of these strategies for all the students.

When this teacher sees the benefit of using these strategies, you may never have to mention them again!

Ok, what else can I do to improve my child's school experience?

Great question.

Many middle and high schools offer non-traditional interesting classes that may be exciting and interesting for your child. They have things like woodworking, shop, salon services, home economics, art. If possible, enroll him in one of these each semester.

This will provide a good change in routine, and will keep him active and engaged.

Make sure his school supplies and materials are organized in a way that he can manage. For example, a 3 ring binder with color coordinated dividers for each class is helpful. One part of the binder, say the front folder, can be for homework, the back cover for finished homework. Have his agenda inside this binder.

Also, a pouch is useful for all his miscellaneous items like pencils, rulers and markers. If his backpack has pockets in it to store items, this can be used as well.

Use several of these strategies at home also. As I said earlier, "when used consistently at home and school, the benefits will be tenfold."

So what if you work with the school and the teacher, you've got your kid organized to the hilt, and it is still not working out?

Unfortunately, this is sometimes the case. I'm not going to lie to you. You might do EVERYTHING I suggested here and more.

But the hard truth is that hard as you try, as great a teacher(s) your child may have, the school he is currently in may not be the best place for him. Maybe it will work out if you wait it out long enough but there are no guarantees.

Keep your options open. Don't rule out public school (I've heard terrible things) or private school (I can't afford it) or home school (are you kidding me?) or a school designed specifically for learning differences (I really can't afford it!)

If the school he's in now, whatever it is, is not working, think about changing it. Don't waste too much precious time. Don't let a school fail your child for 5 years running and then think about making a change.

Look at all your options. Have an open mind. Whatever you decide, be involved, be your child's advocate, use what you learned in this chapter.

School does not have to be a disaster!

Chapter 7

Gifts and Strengths

Key #8: ADD is a gift in disguise.

Ha! Really? I don't think so! A curse, possibly. A gift ... no.

Yes, a gift. I am serious, friend. In the chapter on mindset we talked about your belief system, about having faith in your child, about looking at the positive.

I want you to see the positives in the traits of your child. Maybe you need some help with this one. I know it might seem like a long shot.

The behaviors and characteristics so prevalent in many ADD children are seen in most children. Remember what we talked about when learning what ADD is: the ADD child is a typical child with behaviors and traits magnified 2, 3, or 10 times. Most kids are distractible, stubborn and impulsive, to some degree. With the average child, we don't see these traits as so negative. Stubborn is "strong willed," hyperactive is "energetic."

It's the same with your ADD child! He is more hyperactive, so he's more energetic. He's more stubborn, so he's more persistent. There is nothing wrong with that. In fact, those are gifts that can take him far in life.

Some more examples of "negative" traits that have an accompanying positive trait are:

distractible - curious

forgetful - gets very involved in a task

impulsive - action oriented

inconsistent - flashes of inspiration

Now think about your child. Look through this list. Which traits does your child exhibit? Look at the accompanying positive trait. Can you see it in him?

I get it. I couldn't see it either. Tena was forgetful because she had memory problems; she was distracted because she had focusing problems. I didn't see any positives.

When you start to look for it though, you start to see it. When steered in the right direction, when you harness and nurture these positive traits and channel that energy, each of these will turn out to be a blessing instead of a curse.

Get this in your mind. Knowing that these are not all bad can give you the hope you both need. It will give your child the confidence he needs.

When you call his hyperactivity "energy," when you tell him he is persistent, not stubborn, it heaps a ton of confidence into his otherwise self-doubting head. This is not denial, just a way to look at it differently.

So first, change your mindset. We've talked about mindset at length already. It is ultra-important!

Think good, not bad, positive not negative. Help your child change his mindset too. Focus on the positive and the positive will emerge.

Two great examples of people who harnessed their trait and turned negatives into positives are two phenomenal athletes, Michael Jordan and Michael Phelps. Both of these men have ADD. They learned to channel their energy (hyperactivity) into their sport - one became a superstar basketball player and the other, an all time record Olympic Gold Medal swimmer.

Tena was always easily distracted. But I noticed when she was doing something she loved, she paid attention to it. She didn't notice what was going on around her.

Kids with ADD will concentrate and meditate and focus on something they are really interested in.

Our friend Tyler, whom I have mentioned a few times now, got distracted very easily. But get him started on Minecraft, the online video game, and distractions were virtually non-existent for him. He builds worlds and houses like a pro, and he focuses on that and that only.

This could drive a parent crazy, and the first thought might be "what a waste of time, I have to get him off this thing." If you look closely, though, there just may be some gifts you can help him unwrap.

Pay attention to what your child pays attention to! Minecraft has so many facets to it. Looking at what he likes most about it could tell you something about his interests or talents. You can tell if he is adventurous or resourceful, interested in building, exploration or inventing. Capitalize on it!

If he seems to be an inventor of sorts, get him some books on inventors or really cool inventions, books or movies on new and exciting innovations.

If building and taking things apart on Minecraft is what he loves, he might become a great architect or remodeler of homes, build airplanes or design cars. Possibly he is more the adventurer and explorer ... a paleontologist in the making?

Don't look at your child's obsessions as all negative. There may be a gift in there somewhere that will benefit him now and in the future.

Let's take a look at the trait of distraction, since that is a common thread among most ADD children. An accompanying trait is curious.

Many children with ADD identify with nature and the outdoors. They feel a connection there. You may notice that he looks out the window a lot or his teacher may tell you that he does that at school.

It may seem like he is zoning out, but he could very well be curious about what he sees, wondering how the snow falling stays on the ground or how snow comes about in the first place. He might be listening to the call of a bird and wondering what kind of bird it is.

Ask questions! Find out what he is looking at and what he is thinking. Is he interested in something in particular that he sees or hears outside? Help him to learn more about it, go for a walk out there and explore. Get some books out about it; take him to a museum; take him to the zoo.

Before he goes to school or starts homework, let him spend some time outside. He'll probably focus much better once it's time to come in and get to work.

Find the reason behind his behaviors if you can. Remember I told you about Tyler blurting out that he needs a pencil in class? The rules in that class are that you sharpen your pencil before class starts and you do NOT look in your backpack once class is in session. When his pencil broke, he panicked.

What is the gift or strength? The best way to find out is to ask him.

With Tyler, that is just what his mom did. He answered that he knew the rules and didn't want to break them by searching in his backpack for another pencil. He just panicked and without thinking about it, yelled it out.

The gift or strength is that he wants to follow the rules. But impulsiveness kicked in and the inappropriate blurting resulted.

Take advantage of the teachable moment. Let him know it's ok if his pencil broke or he forgot to sharpen it. Praise him for wanting to follow the rules and wanting to stay out of trouble. That is a good and positive strength Tyler has.

Explain alternative ways of handling the problem. Tell him to count to 5 before he does or says anything. Then let him know he could raise his hand to ask the teacher about getting another pencil.

Explain to his teacher the situation, how he panics when he has a problem and is facing breaking rules. His teacher can suggest alternatives to him as well.

Blurting out in class is not a always a sign of disrespect or of trying to be the class clown. It is sometimes the result of the gift of obedience and wanting to please. Look for that first.

Another trait with a positive bent is inconsistency. Inconsistent - flashes of inspiration.

ADD children often have great imaginations and are wildly ambitious. They will make plans and start projects but never complete them. I can give you a great example of my neighbor Jason I mentioned earlier.

On his 40th birthday, his wife threw a party for him and he gathered everyone around to read a list he made. The list was his goals for the next 10 years. It went something like this:

- Become a youth pastor

- Get my bachelor's degree

- Get my wedding business going

- Have 10 franchises 5 years from now

- Start an online business

- Become an ordained minister and officiate weddings

I cannot even begin to tell you what else was on there. The list was long. I don't remember all of it.

I can tell you this: two years later, only one of these was completed - an ordained minister's license obtained online.

He had some fabulous ideas. Some "flashes of inspiration" in the plans he had.

It is a wonderful gift to be ambitious, creative, imaginative, brilliant. Encourage your child to dream but help him be realistic so he can finish what he starts, and finish well.

What if the opposite is true? He is certainly brilliant or talented in some area(s) but he doesn't want to do anything?

He has such potential but he seems content to stay home and watch TV.

Help him find something he is good at and get him out! He needs to be active and have interests and accomplishments to feed his self-confidence and to expend his energy.

Look for a hobby, look into clubs at school, try some sports. If he's not interested in anything, take him to sporting events, watch some on TV.

When Tena was about 8 years old, she had already taken gymnastics and had been on a swim team for 3 summers.

Then - nothing. She was interested in nothing.

I took her to her little friends' softball games, soccer games, and dance classes. I'd ask her, "Doesn't that look like fun?" She would respond this way every time...

"Yeah, but I don't want to do it."

I can't tell you how frustrating that was!

I even enrolled myself in a hip hop dance class for adults, thinking that watching me would make her want to do it. It didn't. She had a great time watching me humiliate and frustrate myself but she had no interest.

Next, finally, success! I took her to a dance academy down the street and observed a hip hop dance class. She saw some people she knew from school, thought it looked like fun, and I enrolled her that day.

She loved it, and she was good at it. She did it for a couple years, had fun, and she learned a skill. She made some friends and gained confidence.

A Couple Of Other Ways to Discover Your Child's Gifts and Strengths

Watch how your child plays.

How does he relate with other children? What kind of play holds his attention the longest? What does he like to do? Does he like to build, help you cook, draw in the sand? He could be a chef in the making, an artist, a builder.

Is he a "ham" showing off all the time, singing and dancing? It could be he has a gift for entertaining.

Tena is passionate about kids and has been even since she was a kid herself. She babysits all the time, worked at a daycare center, and currently works in the nursery at church. She comes home and tells and re-tells stories about the kids. She is enthusiastic and excited about them. She is drawn to kids like a magnet, and they are drawn to her. She loves to teach them and talk to them. The feeling is mutual – kids love her like crazy.

In Tena's senior year of high school, she changed her career aspirations 4 times. Criminal Justice, Nursing, Real Estate, then ... Early Childhood Education. I think that is the ticket for her. She is a natural.

When I noticed her love for kids, I encouraged her to babysit and every time I had a chance I talked about her to people I knew who might need a sitter. I actually helped get her one of her first babysitting jobs. This passion may end up being a career for Tena, and she will be awesome at it.

Talk to him

We discussed this in the chapter on structure and I encouraged you to talk with your child at bedtime. Do this! Talk with him after school, in the morning at breakfast, whenever you can.

Pay attention to what he talks about.

Ask about his day. What was the best part of the day? How was gym class? Who did you sit with at lunch? As you talk with your child day in and day out, you'll learn more about him.

In the process, you'll probably discover some interests and gifts you didn't even know he had.

Once You Discover His Gifts and Strengths, Write Them Down.

You always want them in the forefront of your mind for several reasons:

1. When you're at the end of your rope, 1 and you think there is nothing your child can do right, it is a valuable reminder.

2. You want to remind him of these gifts to instill confidence in him.

3. You want to constantly help him nurture and develop these gifts.

Keep your list in a safe place. Refer to it often.

Always remember your child has many gifts. Help him to find and use them.

Chapter 8

Lifestyle Changes to Change a Life

Diet

How does diet affect an ADD child?

First, food and diet is never the cause of ADD but it can definitely exacerbate the symptoms. Behavior can easily hinge on what he ate or drank that day.

Artificial substances can negatively affect your child's brain. He may have allergies to some foods or substances contained in certain foods, or just a strong reaction to artificial substances.

It is best to eliminate, or at least greatly reduce your child's intake of refined sugar, white flour, white rice, high fructose corn syrup, aspartame, MSG and nitrates. These have been shown to have adverse effects on many ADD children.

A good test of what affects your child is to eliminate something you think is causing his ADD symptoms to worsen and eliminate that from his diet. After a spaghetti dinner is he more hyper, less focused? Take pasta out of his diet. Whatever the food or ingredient is, remove it.

Observe if there are improvements in his symptoms. Incrementally and slowly bring that substance back into his diet and observe any changes. You will find whether that food significantly affects his behavior or not.

Another tactic to try is eliminating almost everything that could be the culprit, then one by one add foods back in. You might eliminate what I've already mentioned, plus gluten and dairy.

This is very difficult because it's hard to figure out what to feed him!

However, I believe it is one of the most effective ways to determine what does and what does not negatively affect your child's behavior.

If his ADD symptoms significantly lessen while his diet is void of these substances, slowly add one thing back in at a time. Continue for a few days or a week and see if his behavior starts to regress. If not, that food product is probably ok and you can allow that in his diet. If his behavior worsens, take it back out and avoid that food.

Continue until you have tried to add everything back in. You will find what affects him and what doesn't and then adjust his diet accordingly.

The foods we eat can affect our mental health for our benefit or to our detriment. This is true for anyone, but even more so for the ADD child!

Of course, be smart about this. If your child has some medical condition or other reason he needs certain foods, keep them in his diet. His health comes first, so if any of these strategies will be detrimental to his health, please refrain from using them!

Basically, stick with a lot of protein, with more complex carbohydrates (such as vegetables and whole grains), fewer simple carbohydrates (such as candy, potatoes, pasta, bread, cereal) and more Omega-3 fatty acids (such as fish, nuts, olive oil). You will be well on your way to improved brain health for your child.

Make sure he drinks plenty of clean filtered water throughout the day. Not enough water intake can cause dehydration in the brain. Since the brain is about 75% water, this is not a good thing!

Dehydration can cause mental fatigue, decreased cognitive function and mood changes.

What your child needs is more mental strength, enhanced cognitive functioning and balanced moods.

This one simple thing can provide it. How easy is that?

Vitamins

A good multivitamin is important for overall health. Hard as we try to provide our children with a healthy diet, they still don't always get the vitamins and minerals they need. Essential vitamins and minerals are essential for brain health.

That's it! I just wanted to touch on the subject of food and diet. Whole books are written on the subject. I urge you to look into those if you would like more information.

This should give you a good start. Know that what your child puts in his body matters, and it matters a lot.

Sleep

A good night's sleep is essential. Lack of sleep causes difficulty in concentration, memory and can cause emotions to be even more imbalanced.

Be sure to have a regular bedtime for him and stick to it. Even if he's in high school, try to get him to go to bed at a reasonable hour so he gets the sleep he needs.

Most kids need 8-10 hours of sleep per night but it varies depending on age and each individual child.

Some kids have a hard time getting to sleep. They might go to bed at 9 and lay awake until 11.

Insomnia is one of those things that eludes even experts. But there are some simple things to try that may help your child fall asleep faster:

- taking a bath or shower before bed

- reading to him or having him read in bed

- using a sound machine – the sound of the ocean or a babbling brook can soothe a child to sleep

- a cool, not hot bedroom

- make sure they are not hungry but also not full

Exercise

Exercise is not only good for your heart but for your brain!

Exercise provides a nourishing environment for brain cell growth. Cognitive function including memory can improve significantly with exercise.

It has also been shown to be associated with a drop in the stress hormone, helping one to be more emotionally balanced and less stressed throughout the day.

Of course, since your child may have boundless energy, to put it nicely, exercise is a fantastic way for him to get some of that energy worked out so that he is more likely to be able to concentrate and sit still.

It is a great idea to start each day with some physical exercise.

Before school is probably pushing it, but if you can get him doing some jumping jacks, running in place, or jumping rope before school it would be helpful. Do something to get him moving and stimulate that brain. He can get refocused and ready to learn just by doing a little of this every day.

A couple of years ago, Tena got on an exercise kick. She usually does "Insanity," an exercise program on DVD that is intense! It lives up to its name for sure. It incorporates a lot of different moves both standing, squatting and on the ground.

She still does this almost every day, and I can see a tremendous difference, not just in her body but in her brain! She has become much more organized and less scattered in her thinking. Her memory has improved significantly.

I believe much of this improvement is a direct result of regular exercise.

Martial Arts

The general consensus by many experts in the field of child behavior is that the discipline of martial arts will likely lead to improved behavior, self-discipline and self-confidence in children.

One study just blew me away when I read it! It was from an article by Matthew K. Morand, The Effects of Mixed Martial Arts on Behavior of Male Children with Attention Deficit Hyperactivity Disorder.

This was a 12 week study done with male children ages 8-11 all diagnosed with ADHD. All of them participated in a mixed martial arts class. Behavior was monitored according to schoolteachers who completed a behavior checklist throughout the 12 week period. An excerpt from this study:

"Martial Arts was proven to increase percentage of homework completion, academic performance, and percentage of classroom preparation while decreasing the number of classroom rules broken and times inappropriately leaving the seat. This study lends empirical support to martial arts as a positive intervention for children with AD/HD."

Wow - this is impressive!

Martial Arts mixes coordination, movement, discipline, respect for self and others. The results gained from this study are just a natural extension of all of these practices.

Now, I promise you, I am not trying to get you to enroll in the Karen Murphy School of Martial Arts! The extent of my martial arts experience is a self-defense class I took in college about 100 years ago.

I have learned about it over the years, however, by reading up on it and by talking with parents whose children participate in it. I have spoken at length with marital arts instructors and Tena participated in a martial arts class for a year. I have enough confidence in it to say that it is definitely worth a look.

Playing a Musical Instrument

I wasn't sure where this fit into the book. A lifestyle change? Not sure. It's not really a strategy or mindset or anything like that. I almost decided to leave this out.

But I couldn't do it.

It's too important.

Learning to play a musical instrument has amazing benefits in so many areas ranging from academic to social to emotional. Just this one practice can skyrocket your kid's self-confidence, intellectual ability, social adeptness and more.

Many studies have been conducted over the past several decades and they overwhelmingly suggest that this is in fact the case. Some of the benefits that have been discovered that playing an instrument can do:

- Increase memory capacity.

- Help with math skills.

- Improve reading comprehension. Take a look at this excerpt from an impressive study cited in the journal, Psychology of Music: "Children exposed to a multi-year program of music tuition involving training in increasingly complex rhythmic, tonal, and practical skills display superior cognitive performance in reading skills compared with their non-musically trained peers"

- Teach perseverance and self- discipline.

- Enhance listening skills.

- Sharpen concentration.

- Relieve stress

- Promote a sense of accomplishment.

This is just a sampling of some of the benefits. I would have to add another page at least to complete the list!

Learning to play an instrument requires a lot of time, effort and diligence. It requires concentration. It uses eye-hand coordination. The student of music learns tone, pitch and melody. He learns notes and rhythms.

Playing an instrument uses the brain in different ways than just ordinary life and book learning does. I encourage you to explore this avenue as another way to help your child.

Also, I encourage you to engage in some of these lifestyle changes for yourself and other family members as well.

If you all improve your lifestyle, your child will feel like this is just a normal part of life. It will be one less thing that makes him stand out as different. If he is the only one who is exercising and eating a different diet, it will be one more thing that makes him feel different and inferior.

Secondly, a healthier diet, enough rest and regular exercise will improve the health (physical and brain) of all who engage in it. Do this as a favor for the whole family!

Chapter 9

Socially Skilled

"Please don't bring Sam over here anymore. He picks on little Stevie all the time, and he won't listen when I tell him to stop."

"Mom, everyone was invited to Sara's birthday party except me."

I'm sorry but I don't think this Brownie troop is going to work out for Janie. She is just too disruptive."

Have you heard anything like this about your kid? It hurts doesn't it?

Unfortunately, these and similar scenarios are fairly typical in the life of a child with ADD and his family.

Take heart! It doesn't have to be this way. Allow me to shine a bright light into this dismal picture for you!

Key #9: Social skills will naturally improve as a result of implementing the methodologies discussed in this book.

Once you start taking charge and implementing what you've learned, you will notice his social skills improving.

I promise you, I'm not saying we're done and you don't have to work on social skills. I'm also not getting lazy and trying to get out of writing a chapter.

To be honest, though, when you implement what you have learned so far, you will notice a huge change in how your child relates with other people. The quality of his social interactions will have improved dramatically.

Your child is going to make huge strides academically, his level of self-confidence and feelings of self-worth will improve dramatically.

He will have much more control over his behavior and have better communication skills. He won't seem like such a freak to his classmates, neighbors or other family members. He won't feel like he is so different because he won't be so different.

All this will translate into a much healthier and normal social life.

I do understand, however, that even though your child is much better, there may be a little (or more) room for improvement in this area.

It may be necessary to target social skills specifically, and I will share with you some very effective ways to do just that.

Because of the traits many ADD children exhibit, other children don't like to be around them. When they are around them, they often default to teasing and bullying.

Short Simple Steps That Go A Long Way:

Involve your child in groups with people of like interests. Sports teams or clubs that your child enjoys are non-threatening venues where he can be successful in the activity and also connect on the same level with these children.

1. Teach him to quiet himself for 5 seconds before responding to someone or something. This can reduce or prevent instances of "blurting out" and of him voicing inappropriate or inflammatory remarks.

2. Interrupt him to remind him that he just interrupted you. Tell him to let you finish what you were saying. He'll eventually learn the patience to wait until others are finished talking.

3. Practice eye contact with him. Good eye contact is essential for good communication!

4. Make sure he knows and uses basic manners and transitional expressions such as hi and bye, and please and thank you.

5. Tell him about situations in your own life that may be similar to those that are currently plaguing him. This kind of empathy can give him confidence by making him feel more "normal." Also, any solutions you may have come up with could be useful for him as well.

Children, and even adults, may not like being around your child. There are several possibilities of why this is the case. I will be speaking in generalities but some of this may describe your child.

A short attention span and trouble with following directions affects his ability to play games correctly.

- He touches other kids or touches their stuff.

- He can't wait his turn.

- He's too hyper so he irritates other children and can't sit and play quietly.

- He doesn't work well in groups. He tries to take over or doesn't participate at all.

- He doesn't share.

- He doesn't pick up on verbal and non-verbal cues that someone is annoyed so he continues adverse behavior.

- He doesn't understand jokes, plays on words, etc.

- I have seen it firsthand. Tena definitely possessed difficulty with some of these herself.

- Jokes, she missed. Even to this day they often elude her.

- Sharing was not part of her vocabulary.

- She didn't pick up well on verbal and non-verbal cues.

- Let me share with you a great example from about 10 years ago.

We were at a family wedding in Florida, and the day before the wedding we were all playing around in the hotel pool.

Tena was about 8 years old and she was playing in the pool with her uncle and a cousin. At first it was great. I loved watching her play with her relatives, who she only saw once or twice a year, but then I noticed her getting increasingly rambunctious. She was climbing on her uncle's head and his shoulders, splashing him and acting in otherwise obnoxious ways!

My brother told her to stop several times and was starting to get angry, but she did not let up at all.

It got so bad my brother actually started pushing her away and then held her UNDER the water for a couple of seconds trying to make her stop. At one point he yelled to me, "Karen, haven't you taught this kid any control," or something along those lines.

I finally stepped in and made Tena get out of the pool and proceeded to torture her with a long and serious talk about how we play nicely and how we need to listen to and respect others.

Observe your child as he plays and interacts with others

Does he seem oblivious when others are getting annoyed?

Does he get mad and act out if he loses a game?

Does he take his sister's toys and break them in two?

Explain to your child that these behaviors (choose one or two) are part of the reason other children don't want to be with him, that these particular behaviors cause others to become angry, hurt or annoyed. Let him know there are more appropriate responses and behaviors that you and he will be working on.

Punishing him or yelling at him that he did something wrong will not teach him. Your child may not know what he is supposed to do or how he should act.

Role Playing

One of the best teachers is role playing activities. When you are sitting down to dinner or playing a game, model the correct behavior. Point it out to your child. Have him practice it. Do this over and over, for weeks, months, as long as it takes.

Then, when you feel he is getting a grasp on it...

Turn the tables. You display inappropriate behaviors and let him call you out on it. For example, while he is talking, you interrupt and talk over him. While playing a game, you go ahead of him and take your turn when it's his turn.

This will help him develop an awareness of how his behavior affects others. He'll be able to feel what others feel when he does this to them.

You can make it a game. Tell him to call you out whenever you exhibit the inappropriate behavior. Ask him how you should have acted or what you should have done. If he doesn't know, tell him and exhibit the appropriate behavior for him.

This is an excellent way to help your child learn proper behavior and to start learning how to pick up on verbal and non-verbal cues from others.

As you turn the tables and engage in behaviors similar to his default behaviors, he will get annoyed, angry, or hurt. Then he will react in a way that displays his annoyance, anger or hurt. Explain what you've just done, and tell him that the way he is feeling right now is how others feel when he does these things to them.

Eventually he will start to notice cues from people and know when it's time to stop or modify his behavior.

Telling him is one thing, but showing him is another.

"I don't know," you might say. "Isn't that cruel Karen? I don't want to annoy or hurt my kid!"

I say no, it's really not. Taking a turn in front of him or talking over him is not cruel and unusual punishment.

I'll grant you, if you are working on getting him to stop punching other kids, you should forgo turning the tables. I don't want you punching your kid so he can see how it feels. Practice common sense!

Use other people

Other children can be excellent role models for him as well. You can always point out behavior in others that you would like him to emulate. Heed this warning however:

Be careful how you do this and how often. You don't want to continually "compare" your child to someone else. Repeatedly telling him something like, "look at your sister, she stays in her seat at dinner " or "look at Matt, he shares his toys." can build resentment in him toward that person.

You be the judge. If you see resentment building, or some other negative feelings that may cause this to backfire, ease up on using others as models.

As long as he sees real live examples, it will help him get those behavior patterns ingrained in his brain, and he will start behaving that way himself.

You can also use movies and television as examples. As you watch with him, talk with him about how a character(s) acted or reacted in a certain situation that was praiseworthy. It may be hard to find anything in today's media, but it's there!

Of course, the opposite is out there, and it's probably a lot more plentiful. It's best to be careful about what your child watches. Seeing impulsive and irresponsible behavior constantly on TV (and it's everywhere on the air waves) will only exacerbate those behaviors in him. He'll see it as normal, he'll think it and before long he'll do it.

A few years ago, we got rid of TV. We have no cable, no satellite dish, nothing but Netflix. We can watch several shows that are streamed through our Roku box onto our television screen. One show that Tena has been hooked on for the last 3 years is the Dick Van Dyke show.

If you haven't been around as long as I have, you may not be familiar with it. Dick Van Dyke was originally aired in the early 1960's and ran for about 5 years. It's about a family of 3 where Dad (Dick Van Dyke) is a comedy writer and Mom (Mary Tyler Moore) is a housewife, and they have one son.

In my opinion, the show is loaded with clever humor. I'm hooked on it too, but the best part is the good old fashioned morals and values exhibited throughout each episode. Whenever impulsive behavior or "wrong" behavior occurs, it is recognized and resolved before the end of each episode. I think shows like this are great teachers. I love that Tena watches this, even now at 19. Look for shows like this and discuss with your child these positive ways of handling situations.

Keep Track

It's always a good idea to use a chart even for teaching social behavior, similar to one you use for chores or schedule. Write the behavior down and when you "catch him being good" as they say, mark the chart.

Have it understood from the beginning that after so many checks (or tokens or whatever works for you both) are attained, he gets some type of reward or privilege.

Always praise him for the proper behavior! Then mark his chart. Reinforce, Reinforce, Reinforce.

Play Dates - Preparation and Intervention

Having children over is a fantastic way to observe and teach your child proper social behavior. Try to have children over for play dates on a regular basis. If your child doesn't have friends right now, invite cousins or neighbors if possible.

BEFORE little guests come, prepare your child!

Go over the behaviors you are targeting with him. Make sure he remembers the one or two things he needs to focus on as he interacts with these children.

Remind him of his chart and your reward system.

As you observe, when you see him engaging in the "wrong" behavior, call him aside. DO NOT; I repeat, DO NOT, correct him in front of his friends!

Ask him if he knows why you called him out. If not, tell him yourself and be sure he knows what the appropriate behavior or response should have been. Let him go back to his friends.

If the behavior is too out of control and he is not correcting it, you may have to cut play dates short.

As you follow these methods repeatedly, his interaction with others will improve.

Language - Play on Words

Another obstacle to your child's acceptance in the social community is language and communication issues. I mentioned that children with ADD often do not understand word play, and thus do not "get" jokes or sarcasm.

Now, if your child doesn't have this problem, this may seem silly or of minimal importance, but truly many ADD kids suffer from this.

Inability to understand jokes, sarcasm or stories with a twist can impede the ability to communicate well with others and can make a child, smart as he may be, feel and look stupid.

So, what to do? If you will remember from a previous chapter, I stressed the importance of reading. This is imperative! The more you read to him the better he understands language. The better he understands language, the better he will understand humor.

I'm talking about reading in general. Use any books you want him to read or you want to read to him.

You may find, however, that he needs more than that. Nothing wrong with deliberately selected reading to help him specifically in this area.

Joke books are a great tool. Find a book with a lot of humor in it that you know he may not understand. Just go through the book and whatever he doesn't understand, explain it. Little by little, his mind will be able to find its way to wrapping itself around this type of humor and use of language.

When Tena was young, we read a lot of Amelia Bedila books. Amelia constantly misunderstood instructions and took things so literally that she was always messing up. They are funny books, but they also teach how words and phrases have many different meanings. Tena learned a lot of these words and phrases through these books.

When I talk, I use a lot of idioms. Many people do. "A dime a dozen, saved by the bell, mum's the word." These convey a message in a unique way. There are literally hundreds of idioms, and many are very, very common in the English language, but your child doesn't know or understand them.

Tena still gives me that quizzical look when I spout some of these little sayings. Some were just more common from my time (the olden days) so she hasn't heard them much. However, many are still used today in everyday speech by everyday people, and your child will do well to understand them.

These are actually fun to learn because they sound so silly and nonsensical. Practice these together.

Try choosing two and find ways to use them often when speaking with him. For example, talk about how good he is at something and how it's a "piece of cake" for him. See if he can figure out what "piece of cake" means. Let him do the same with you.

Blunt or Just Plain Rude?

You gotta love kids. They say what's on their mind and ask tons of questions. However, when your kid is 10, 12 or 18, saying what's on his mind can go from cute to downright rude. Just another reason some kids might avoid yours like the plague!

I have a daughter who is about a year and a half younger than Tena. Sarah does not have ADD but many of her remarks, and her habit of speaking before thinking, are reminiscent of what you might hear from some ADD children. They serve as great examples for this topic, and I suspect many of you have had an experience like this one:

At dinner, "This chicken is disgusting."

When getting into my car, "it stinks in here."

My clothes: "Where did you get that? That's an old lady sweater."

Ouch. Even coming from a 12 year old it hurts!

How should you respond?

Let's go back to my disgusting chicken. In response to her comment, I said something like, "that was rude." The conversation continued like this, with the tone of voice impatient and rude on both sides.

Sarah: Well, I don't like it.

Me: Then don't eat it.

Sarah: What am I supposed to eat?

Me: I don't care. Make Ramen.

Sarah: I don't want Ramen. I had Ramen for lunch.

Me: Then don't eat! Go to your room and don't come back until you can apologize and act civil!

This was not productive - I do not recommend this kind of discussion!

A better chicken scenario would have gone like this:

Sarah: This chicken is disgusting.

Me: You don't have to like it, but it makes me feel bad when you tell me something I made is disgusting.

Sarah: Well, I don't want it. What am I supposed to eat?

Me: First we're going to figure out a better way you could have said that you don't like the chicken.

Then, I could have asked her how she might have said it differently and even give some ideas of my own:

Eat it anyway and don't complain.

Say, "I'm sorry Mom, but I don't like this, can I have something else?"

Either of these would have been better and would have helped us avoid a "chicken fight."

It's important to note that no matter what is said, don't get angry - TEACH!

As you hear about your child blurting out things like this with classmates, or if you observe him doing this yourself, take advantage of it and teach him better ways to communicate his opinions or when it might be more appropriate to keep his opinions to himself.

Misinterpretations

Children with ADD often misinterpret the meaning of others' actions towards them.

Somebody rushes off from them because they are late for class and your child interprets that this kid doesn't like him.

His teacher corrects him and he automatically assumes the teacher must think he's stupid.

Treat this like you would his inappropriate comments to others. When you hear or observe that your child is misinterpreting others' behaviors toward him, TEACH.

Help him figure out reasons why someone may have acted the way they did.

Your child will believe and assume one thing and one thing only. He can't see any other reason behind it. This causes him more anxiety and more feelings of inferiority. It stifles that self-confidence that otherwise might be getting stronger.

It must be addressed.

As you address these misinterpretations, he will begin to learn that it's not always about him. It's not always that someone is mad at him. It doesn't always mean he messed up...again.

Be aware of your child and how he interprets things that happen around him or that happen to him. Keep the communication open and help him to see things as they really are.

Your child can have a healthy social life. Be consistent and deliberate. You won't be disappointed.

Chapter 10

I Need More! Getting Outside Help

Key #10: You are not a failure if you need other outside interventions. Get outside help if you need it!

You have ingested a ton of invaluable information in these last nine chapters. I hope you will begin to implement some of these ideas immediately.

But I'll be honest with your here. Sometimes it takes more. You're going to see tremendous improvement, but depending on the severity of your child's symptoms, more is sometimes needed. What you can do yourself is not always enough.

That's ok.

In this chapter we'll explore other options, outside interventions that may be the perfect fit for your child's needs.

Natural Remedies

We've talked a little bit about lifestyle changes, including changes in diet. But in addition to just diet change, supplementation with natural products can be very helpful to the ADD child. Neurotransmitters in the brain are responsible for different areas of the brain to "connect" and talk to each other. People with ADD often have a deficiency in one or more of these neurotransmitters.

Fatty acids are used to make two neurotransmitters, dopamine and norepinephrine. Since our bodies cannot make fatty acids, they must come from food sources like fish, nuts and canola oil. But people, especially children, do not get enough of these types of foods. It can be almost impossible to get a kid to eat more fish and nuts!

Great news: Supplements.

Fish oil supplements are a wonderful source of fatty acids. If your child can't tolerate or is allergic to fish, there are other oils out there that come from seeds and nuts and are excellent sources of fatty acids as well, such as black current or flax seed oil.

Another very useful and effective supplement is zinc , Zinc aids in the production of two of the neurotransmitters and also contributes to the metabolism of fatty acids. So, even fatty acid intake in small amounts can be used by the body more effectively when zinc is added to the diet.

As always, I recommend consulting your doctor before starting a regimen of any supplementation. Be careful about mixing natural remedies with certain medications. Always take precaution and work closely with your doctor.

Note: Some doctors do not believe in, or have much faith in natural remedies. They will discourage you from using any natural supplements and/or will know very little about them.

Find a medical doctor who is open to and knowledgeable about both, and work closely with him or her.

ADHD coaching

ADHD coaching is a fairly new, but rigorously growing profession as the need for help for people with ADD continues to rise. Coaches work one on one with clients to help them learn and understand their strengths and weaknesses and to develop strategies to overcome those weaknesses and maximize their abilities.

Coaches work closely with clients to help them identify changes they would like to make and provide ongoing support and help in making those changes. They provide feedback, encouragement, recommendations, strategies and techniques to fit each client and will monitor the client's progress to help them stay on track. An ADD coach can create structure and organization out of chaos and confusion, by simplifying the client's life using practical and concrete tools for organization and time management. The support, encouragement and practical help gained by the use of an ADD coach can be a monumental benefit to any child or adult with ADD.

To find a coach and for more information, go to http://www.adhdcoaches.org/

Learning RX

As my husband and I were agonizing over how to help Tena with her reading, two of Scott's sisters recommended Learning RX. Both of them had daughters (with ADD) who completed the program in Little Rock, Arkansas. One of his sisters lived about 3 hours from there, but they made the trek twice a week. Both of these girls had amazing success and their parents raved about the difference it made in their daughters' abilities and achievements. We decided it was worth a look.

We found that in the near future, the first center would be opening in a nearby town in Georgia. Answered prayer! We signed Tena up, and she was the first student of the first and only center in our state. We actually met in the director's home for the first several months!

Tena did the reading program when she was 10, and Math RX her freshman year in high school.

So what is it?

Learning Rx was founded in 1986 by Dr. Ken Gibson and other professionals in Appleton, Wisconsin. It is a brain training program, much different than tutoring and many times more effective.

Students of this program will engage in interactive exercises that will force them to focus and use their brain in ways that strengthen and grow neuronal connections.

Through a series of brain training exercises, students' cognitive abilities are significantly increased. Improvements in processing speed, reasoning, memory and attention are a direct result of the training.

Learning RX was expensive, but it was worth it in Tena's case and may work for your child.

One of Tena's weaknesses was her working memory. She could do a math problem and before she got her answer down on paper it already left her head.

Careless mistakes abounded as well.

Two or three step math problems? Forget about it!

It was incredibly frustrating because I knew she could do these problems, but because of her memory, the evidence couldn't be seen on paper.

After just a few weeks of Math RX, Tena was improving dramatically. She was in Algebra 1 - Algebra does not exactly consist of one step problems! Some were 3, 4, 5 steps, with negative numbers and variables everywhere...it was overwhelming even to me.

But her focus was stronger and the working memory much improved. From brain to paper became a "no brainer." Tena ended up with a 96 in the class.

Medication

This is a tough one for most parents and it was a very real dilemma for me. I will not tell you that you must absolutely avoid medication. It has been effective for many children with ADD and those who once suffered with severe symptoms have enjoyed "normalcy" and success.

I will say this: please view medication as a temporary solution. Use it in conjunction with the methods and strategies you learned from earlier chapters and whatever other methodologies you want to try or have already found to be helpful.

Do NOT depend on medications to "solve" the problems your child is experiencing.

You want him to be able to learn the strategies that will lead him to success in his adult years. Leaning on medication will only make him dependent on it. No one should stay on a medication forever if they can help it, and if the time comes when you want to decrease or eliminate his medication, your child needs to have the skills necessary to live a productive adult life without it.

It's hard work to teach and train and strategize - but it is well worth it. Your child will thank you for it one day.

Let's say you've decided to try medication. Something needs to be done immediately.

Be proactive with medication use. When your doctor prescribes a medication for your child, do your own research! Find out everything you can about it: What's in it? What could be long term effects, risks and side effects? Would the benefits outweigh the risk?

Some common side effects of many of the stimulant medications are lack of sleep, loss of appetite, "spacing out," and headaches, to name a few. Your child may or may not experience these but you have to carefully consider this when making your decision.

Determine exactly what you hope to see improve; have a checklist, then monitor your child closely. Have his teacher(s) do the same. If it's not helping or helping "too much" (maybe instead of being hyper your child is now a zombie), work with your doctor to change the dosage or possibly try a different medication.

Remember: engage in a comprehensive program to assist your child. Don't depend solely on medication. It is NOT a cure and implementing strategies, therapies, changes in lifestyle, etc. can eventually reduce or even eliminate the need for meds altogether.

What Else?

There is an amazing amount of help available out there. I cannot begin to describe all of it in this one little book, but I do encourage you to investigate everything you can possibly find. Consider what I have outlined in this chapter. Also, you may want to try other avenues to help your child.

Start with the list below. Some of these may be more than you need for your child's particular situation and symptoms, but some may be just what you need. Look these up and decide what you think will work for your child. Start on the web and go from there. If you discover more than is on this list, by all means, check it out!

counseling

psychotherapy

family therapy

speech and language pathology

Neurofeedback

art therapy

music therapy

Brain Gym

integrated listening (iLs)

Now that you have a strong base of ideas and strategies to bring success into the life of your child, it's time to get started!

Take it one step at a time. Do what you both can handle. Keep using what works and don't spend time and energy on what doesn't.

Will you make mistakes? Of course you will. Learn from them and go on. Do your best. There is no doubt - your child WILL benefit.

One last thing...

Enjoy your journey. And love watching your child achieve stellar success in school, at home, in life!

Bonus Chapter:

Homework Tips

Homework can be harder than normal for a child with ADD. Try these tips and tricks and watch homework time become more productive, less frustrating, and less time consuming for both you and your child!

First, let's look at how to prevent some of the initial frustration your child may have from the get-go, then get into some specific strategies.

A lot of homework frustration is due to forgetting what he learned in class just days or less after he learned it. His homework might as well be a page out of a nuclear physics textbook as foreign as it looks to him.

This is true for many people. In fact, countless studies have shown that without review, most of what is learned is lost within just a couple of days. Astonishingly enough, a study of college students once showed that, only days after a lecture (without reviewing afterwards), most students had forgotten about 90% of what they learned!

When your child comes home from school, try to take about 15 minutes to review what he learned that day. Look at his notes, his handouts, his textbook. The best time to review materials is within a day or two after the material has been read or presented.

It may seem like a waste of time. You feel a need to get immediately to his homework because it can take so darn long and you have no time to waste! But no worries about that. As you do this review on a regular basis, you will see homework become easier and preparation for tests a breeze compared to before.

Make it Worth His While

Children with ADD often have a hard time connecting future events, like connecting a future grade on a report card with the homework he is doing today. Use charts and checklists to mark his progress and create immediate rewards. For example, when he succeeds at working for 15 minutes straight, give him a break with a favorite snack or give points that will add up throughout homework time to achieve some reward or privilege at the end of that time. When or how often you reward will all depend on how long he can wait without losing the mental connection between the work and the reward.

Be Ready with the Right Mindset.

Understand that children with ADD require more monitoring and more patience than a non-ADD child. In most cases you will have to provide assistance with homework and it could be a long haul. Be mentally prepared for it and it will go more smoothly for both of you.

Ok, let's get down to some specifics!

You're sitting down to get the homework done:

- Make sure all supplies are readily available. Create a homework supplies box that has everything he may need and is only used at homework time.

- Remove distractions. Move away from the window or close the blinds or curtains. Move him away from little brother who is watching TV or from the dog who's begging for his snack.

- Have him work near you so that you can monitor him and so that you are available to him for help and he doesn't have to seek you out.

- Catch up on your own paperwork during homework time – pay bills, balance your checkbook, send emails. This helps you to take advantage of the time and also sets an example for your child of how to sit and focus on a task.

- Do homework at the same time every day. If sports and activities get in the way, be as consistent as possible. Maybe homework is 4:00 on non-activity days, 7:00 on activity days.

- Start with a harder subject. Weariness and frustration can grow with every minute. It's best to have easier work to do near the end.

- Take breaks when he needs them, even if it's every 5 minutes. For him to go into a tailspin is not conducive to learning! Let him get away from it when he needs to.

- Shift from one subject to the next if one is getting too frustrating or taking too long. Give him a few minutes to adjust to the change, and then dive in.

- Let him fuel his brain with healthy snacks in the middle of his homework time. Make sure he drinks plenty of water. Well-hydrated and fuel-filled brain cells can improve thinking and performance!

- Give him time. Children with ADD often take longer to process information.

- Check with his teacher to see if he can do a lesser amount of work if it is too much for him. When my daughter was in 4th grade, we worked it out where she would do every other math problem.

- To help him learn vocabulary words or do other memorizing, read and record definitions or questions/answers first, instead of writing. Have him write them down later.

- Make sure he understands the directions. After reading them, have him repeat them in his own words.

- After answering a question, have him look back at the question to make sure he answered exactly to what was asked. Develop this as a habit. It will help in school, on tests, and SAT and ACT exams in the future.

- If he is "zoning out."

Ask him what he is thinking about. Many children with ADD think differently and perceive the world very differently than other kids. They are very curious about nature and their surroundings... how things work, why something happens the way it does. You might find he is wondering about what how the clock hands know to move the way they do, or what kind of bird is making that cool sound outside.

If his mind is wandering in this direction, talk about it for a minute and try to answer his questions. Google it quickly and satisfy his curiosity. Go outside for a few minutes and try to find the bird making that sound. Now he's had his questions answered and he will be better able to focus on the task at hand.

- Allow him to listen to music, return a few text messages, or play with play dough or a stress ball. Often these "distractions" help a child with ADD to focus on his work. These seem counterproductive, but give them a try. You may be surprised.

- Use movement and hands on methods utilizing a couple (or more) of his senses. Some things you can have him do:

* Jump rope while spelling words to the beat of each jump.

Sit on an exercise ball while studying - the movement helps the hyperactive child to be able to move around but still look at his work.

* Walk around inside or outside the house while memorizing.

* Throw a ball back and forth doing questions and answers to study for a test.

* Use play dough, shaving cream, or whipped cream to write out spelling words.

* Use a calculator, not for calculating but for touching the numbers he is working with.

* Find pictures and photos about what he is studying. It makes it come to life and will grab his attention. When my daughter had to do a project on hydras (a close relative of the coral and jellyfish), we were both fascinated watching a YouTube video of how this polyp stings and eats its prey. A tedious science project that we both hated turned into an adventure!

Using your hands and engaging the senses not only makes homework and learning more fun, but it also aids in comprehension, retention and attention.

Just be creative. Or if you're like me (not a creative bone in your body), go online. You'll find plenty of help on the web.

Don't worry about the extra time it takes! Just like the review you will be doing every day, it will take some time but it will pay off in the end.

Strategies for Specific Subjects

Reading

Reading can be so overwhelming. Too many words on a page, words too close together, comprehension problems. Try these simple ideas:

- If reading homework requires answering questions at the end, try having him read the questions first.

- Take turns reading. Let him read a few sentences or a paragraph, then you read. This takes the pressure off.

- Use a ruler or colored paper to cover up the text underneath the line he is reading. This removes the stress of seeing the whole page and keeps him from losing his place.

- Have him read out loud or whisper while reading. Often comprehension improves using this method.

- Have him act out stories, read w/inflection and enthusiasm. You can do this with him, or just model it for him as you read to him.

- Have him interact with the text he is reading. For example, he reads a few sentences or a paragraph, and then writes a "title" or main idea he got from the text. Once finished, he re-reads the whole thing. He, with your help if he needs it, figures out main idea(s) of the entire text he has read.

- Second time around reading something, have him circle unknown words. Then let him try to figure out meaning from context first, then look words up.

- Use audio books. Many textbooks are in this form now, as well as many novels. Listening often aids in comprehension and helps to learn pronunciation. He can read along or not, whichever works best. You can find many of these online for free. You can also read out loud to him if you don't have or don't want to use an audio book.

Writing

- Use wide ruled notepaper.

- Have him write on every other line.

- Brainstorm with him and write down the ideas. Let him write or draw them if he wants to. Don't worry about grammar or spelling in brainstorming sessions.

- When beginning to write, if he is stuck, ask questions. Look over the ideas from your brainstorming session and ask how he might start his first sentence. If he doesn't know, give him one and ask him to say it in his own words.

- Type as he talks because when it comes down to his writing what he said, he may already have forgotten it.

- Help him organize his ideas. Have him write ideas on individual index cards and help him group those that should go together when writing the paper.

- Use graphic organizers to structure writing projects. These will help him to organize his thoughts logically before putting pen to paper. Many different organizers can be found online. One good source: http://www.eduplace.com/graphicorganizer

Math

- use M&Ms, an abacus, dice or some other manipulative for counting, adding and subtracting.

- Use playing cards to practice operations with negatives and positives (make one of the colors negatives, the other positives)

- Use graph paper for long problems like multiplication and long division. This will help him keep numbers in the proper rows and columns to reduce confusion.

- Draw a box around each math problem on his paper. This way, each problem has its own defined space so numbers are not written all over the place and problems won't get mixed up.

- Have him develop a habit of looking at his final answer to a problem before continuing. Common simple mistakes like forgetting to put a negative sign in front of a number or leaving out a variable yields a wrong answer!

- Teach acronyms to remember math rules and concepts. For example, BEDMAS is an acronym for sequence in handling math problems-brackets, exponents, division, multiplication, addition, subtraction.

- Take one step at a time. Please don't be overwhelmed by all of this! Little by little, you will begin to enjoy homework time with your child. It's precious time you get to spend together that one day will be gone. Make this precious time quality time, to be dreaded and feared no longer!

I would love to hear from you regarding any successes you have had using what you've learned from this book and also any outside help you have tried. Any suggestions and constructive criticisms are also welcome!

I want to provide as much encouragement and useful information as possible to my readers, and as I acquire feedback from you, will definitely add any helpful information to future updates of the book.

You can contact me at kstgmurf@gmail.com.

Resources

Organizations:

CHADD (Children and Adults with Attention-Deficit/Hyperactivity Disorder)

http://www.chadd.org/

ADDA (Attention Deficit Disorder Organization)
http://www.add.org/

The Hyperactive Children's Support Group http://www.hacsg.org.uk/

LDA (Learning Disabilities Association of America
http://www.ldanatl.org/

Yahoo groups:

ADD-ADHD-parents

ADD-ADHD

adultadd

Some excellent schools that specialize in working with children with learning differences and learning disabilities:

Near Boston: http://www.landmarkschool.org/ Landmark school

Near Boston: http://www.carrollschool.org/ Carroll school

Dallas, TX: http://www.shelton.org/ Shelton school

Near Nashville, TN: http://curreyingram.org/ Currey Ingram Academy

Traverse City, MI: http://www.leelanau.org/ Leelanau school

Potterville, NJ: http://www.purnell.org/ Purnell school

Most of you probably don't live near any of these schools. Visit the web and search schools for learning disabilities, learning differences, ADHD, etc. More are popping up everywhere and you may find one of interest that is close enough to you.

Bibliography

Aamod, Sandra, Ph.D & Wang, Sam Ph.D, Welcome to Your Child's Brain, New York: Bloomsburg, 2011. Print.

"ADHD and Art Therapy." Art for the Mind, Body and Soul: Art Therapy as an Alternative Way to Help You. Longwood University. 30 Mar. 2012. Web. 23 Jul. 2013

ADHD in Children Health Center. "Impulse Control: Managing Behaviors of ADHD Kids." WebMD. N.p.n.d. Web. 16 Jun. 2013.

Archer, Dale, Better than Normal. New York: The Penguin Group, 2009. Print.

Bailey, Eileen. Ten Suggestions for Winning the Homework Wars. HealthCentral. N.p. healthcentral.com 27 jun. 2011. Web. 28 Jul. 2013.

Barkley, Russell A., Ph.D., Taking Charge of ADHD: The Complete Authoritative Guide for Parents. New York: The Guilford Press, 2000. Print.

Brain Spade Team. "Top 7 Brain Benefits of Drinking Water." brain spade Grow Your Brain. 18 May 2013. Web. 13 Aug. 2013

Chelonian, Lisa. "Can Music Education Enhance Brain Functioning and Academic Learning?" Brain Connection. Posit Science Corporation. 15 May 2000. Web. 29 Jul 2013

Conners, Valerie. "Can playing a musical instrument make you smarter?" Discovery, N.p.n.d. Web. 23 Jul. 2013.

Converse, Judy, MPH, RD, LD., Special Needs Kids Eat Right. New York: The Penguin Group, 2009. Print.

Corman, Catherine A., & Hallowell, Edward M., M.D., Positively ADD: Real Success Stories to Inspire your Dreams. New York: Walker Publishing Co., Inc., 2006. Print.

Formica, Michael J. "Martial Arts and ADD/ADHD." Psychology Today. Enlightened Living. 07 Jul. 2008. Web. 23 Jul. 2013

Greene, Ross W., Ph.D., The Explosive Child: A New Approach for Understanding and Parenting Easily Frustrated, "Chronically inflexible" Children. New York: HarperCollins Publishers, 2005. Print.

Hallowell, Edward M., M.D.& Ratey, John J., M.D., Driven to Distraction: Recognizing and Coping with Attention Deficit Disorder from Childhood Through Adulthood. New York: Simon & Schuster. 1995. Print.

Hallowell, Edward M., M.D. & Jensen, Peter S., M.D., Superparenting for ADD. New York: Ballentine Books, 2010. Print.

Matthews, Michael. "18 Benefits of Playing a Musical Instrument." Effective Music Teaching. Music Advocacy, 28 Aug. 2011. Web. 23 Jul. 2013.

Morand, Matthew K. "The Effects of Mixed Martial Arts on Behavior of Male Children with Attention Deficit Hyperactivity Disorder." Diss. Hofstra University, 2004. Print. "Diagnosing ADD/ADHD." Your ADHD Online Newsletter. 2013. Web. 14 Jun. 2013.

Taylor, John F., The Survival Guide for Kids with ADD or ADHD. Minneapolis: Free Spirit Publishing, Inc., 2006. Print.

Taylor, Kate. "Get the ADHD Facts You Need to Help Your Child: Top 11 ADHD Myths and Facts." Lifescript, Healthy Living for Women. 11 Oct. 2013. Web. 01 May 2013.

Walker, Beth, The Girls Guide to ADHD: Don't Lose this Book! Bethesda: Woodbine House Inc., 2005. Print.

Zeigler Dendy, Chris A., Teenagers with ADD and ADHD: A Guide for Parents and Professionals. Bethesda: Woodbine House, Inc., 2006. Print.

Interview with Andrea Cheetham, former Interrelated Exceptional Education Teacher and Exceptional Education Department Chair.

Interviews with parents of ADHD children including Robyn McDevitt whose son is featured in this book.

Made in the USA
Lexington, KY
08 January 2015